DYNAMIC POSTURE AND CONDITIONING FOR WOMEN

Mary Jo Reiter
University of Utah

Nancy Cato
University of Minnesota

Illustrated by
Mary Ann Bayless

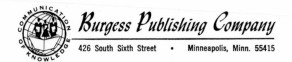
Burgess Publishing Company

426 South Sixth Street • Minneapolis, Minn. 55415

PHYSICAL EDUCATION CONSULTANT TO THE PUBLISHER:

Eloise M. Jaeger
Chairman, Department of Physical Education for Women
University of Minnesota

FOREWORD

Today millions of people are becoming increasingly aware of the importance of exercise and conditioning as a part of their daily lives and are fast moving from the role of spectator to one of active participant. The value of exercise programs as related to appearance, general well-being and work output for the average individual is a well established fact. Consequently, the desire on the part of many individuals to better understand the functioning of the human body and to plan and carry out an intelligent program has never been greater or more needed.

DYNAMIC POSTURE AND CONDITIONING represents a fresh, challenging, and informative approach to this subject for the college student. Much has been written about posture and conditioning in general but the authors of this text have gone well beyond the concepts usually expressed. This approach is unique not only in that it interrelates conditioning with posture but that it treats specific conditioning as related to specific physical concerns and sports skills and exercise for specific needs. Flexibility, relaxation, mobility, weight management, menstruation and dysmenorrhea are some of the common problems discussed. In addition, posture as an active and operative part of the life of the human being is dealt with in a complete and scientific manner.

Those individuals who study and apply the material contained in this book will not only enhance their physical and psychological sense of well-being but will become more sensitive to the way in which they perceive their own bodies and body movement.

Eloise M. Jaeger
University of Minnesota

PREFACE

This book is an outgrowth of the authors' belief that one of the most prominent threats to an affluent society takes root in its complacency with respect to man's fundamental need for vigorous and efficient use of the human body. Such a society is too often willing to relinquish the rewards inherent in consistent, strenuous exercise and too frequently prone to settle for the spoils which inevitably result from overindulgent, sedentary living. Evidence of this fact envelops us: wholesale indifference to the need for regularity in exercise, absence of common concern for efficiency in movement, the tendency to demonstrate only periodical concern for tension reduction, and, finally, dietary habits which are both vacillating and unconstrained. A dichotomy seems to exist. On the one hand society devotes its finest minds and most elaborate equipment to medical research designed to prevent disease, discover new cures, and increase longevity. Yet this same society invents and subsequently lavishes on its people a myriad of labor-saving devices which propagate physical idleness and ineffective use and care of the human body.

It should be quite clear that education for efficient posture and conditioning is an eminently worthwhile if not absolutely essential prerequisite for dynamic living in today's world. Hopefully, this book will help to meet that educational need. The authors believe that habits derive from attitudes which are, in turn, influenced by the knowledge, understanding, and appreciation one possesses. This book seeks to present practical, scientifically sound knowledge in a very personal style and in nontechnical language. It proposes to be interesting, stimulating, challenging, and motivating. It will probably be as effective as the reader is serious about understanding the content and implementing the recommended exercises and patterns for efficient movement.

The book is designed as a basic text for general college classes dealing with posture and conditioning. It should be equally suitable for the general adult reader seeking a personal plan for improving physical efficiency both at work and at play. Portions of the book may be appropriate for use with high school students, while other sections may be used effectively in professional college classes.

The authors are indebted to students and professional colleagues who have questioned, discussed, encouraged, and thereby contributed many ideas and considerable motivation for the initial undertaking and the completion of this book. Special and individual appreciation is expressed to Jeralyn Plack for typing the manuscript and to Julie Paulson, College Editor at Burgess Publishing Company, whom death claimed before our work was complete.

Nancy Cato
Mary Jo Reiter

CONTENTS

Part I – Conditioning

Chapter   Page

Part I

CONDITIONING

Chapter 1

INTRODUCTION

In the pursuit of living, in the search for an active, abundant, and extended life you are often limited by a single self-imposed handicap—the poor physical condition of your body. It seems important to understand that your appearance and your capacity for work and play are largely determined by the physical condition of your body. And the physical condition of your body is, in turn, directly influenced by the amount and kinds of exercise required of it, the nutrition furnished it, and the rest and relaxation granted it. In other words, your capacity for optimal daily living is either enhanced or limited by the physical efficiency of your body. This is precisely why you must be concerned about conditioning. You have often read or heard people speak about physical exercise programs. The term "physical exercise" is a very general one which implies some type of bodily activity, performance or exertion, and when considered in these terms, you perform exercise every day of your life. Thus, when you read of an "exercise program" the reference seems vague and general. It doesn't clearly identify the reason for doing the exercising. Therefore, this book will seek to develop the concept of conditioning programs rather than exercise programs.

The Dynamic Conditioning Program

The dynamic conditioning concept should be viewed as having two basic dimensions: general and specific. The general or "overall" conditioning program is basic to all others; it is the only lasting foundation on which to build subsequent, more specific conditioning programs. The general conditioning refers to developing and maintaining a level of strength, flexibility, and endurance which enables you to maintain an erect alignment, complete your work, participate in active recreation, and, having done all, to possess a reserve supply of energy.

1

The specific conditioning refers to programs which seek to develop the physical capacities required for successful performance in selected activities. Some sports and recreational activities require specific conditioning emphasis. For example, skiing may require more leg strength than your general, basic conditioning program develops. Hence, unless you engage in a specific skiing conditioning program prior to taking skiing instruction, you may greatly handicap the ability of your body to perform the basic skills required to ski. Specific muscle groups must already have sufficient strength and endurance to do the work required of them in the performance of skiing skills. Thus, a ski conditioning program is the means by which you attain the strength, the mobility, the balance, and the endurance level necessary to be able to put your understanding of how to perform a skiing skill into action.

It seems quite possible that many beginning and novice performers become unnecessarily discouraged and disappointed while trying to learn sport skills simply because they are not physically ready to learn. When we consider the acknowledged importance of one's readiness to learn, the concept herein promoted may, for many individuals, be the key to the door of successful and satisfying performance.

Since you are constantly adapting to your environment, it is essential to view both general and specific body conditioning needs as changing needs. Continuous evaluation of personal conditioning needs calls for a concept of dynamic body conditioning.

Dynamic Conditioning—A Self-directed Effort

Your body can be weak, slumped, and ill-shaped at twenty-two or you can have a strong, erect, well-proportioned body at fifty-two. Which body you have is your choice. An objective look at the reflection of your body in a mirror and an unbiased assessment of your energy reserve will tell you in an instant how "old" your body is in terms of appearance and function. It is interesting to note that you first attended to brushing your teeth, bathing, and caring for your hair because these tasks were imposed on you. Gradually they became habits and it wasn't until much later that you realized their importance to your health and appearance. Undoubtedly some of you already realize the importance of conditioning and are anxious to begin. Others may be less enthusiastic. If you find it necessary, "impose" the conditioning program on yourself. Let it become habit and eventually, through experience, you will begin to realize its importance. Since the significance that you attach to an effort largely determines your faithfulness in seeing it through to the finish, you have to determine that the effort you devote to this program will be consistent daily. No conditioning program can succeed if you bring to it only sporadic interest and effort.

There is no "best" time of day appropriate for everyone intending to follow a conditioning program. You may either select a time that is most practical in your schedule or you may let your temperament decide. If exercise relaxes you, do it just prior to your bath or just before you retire for the day. If you find exercise stimulating, get up a few minutes early and start your day this way. In any case, do not make the mistake of rationalizing the time issue. A compromising attitude will keep you from achieving your goal. It would be dishonest to submit that you do not have fifteen minutes daily to devote to a body conditioning program. Your conditioning program will be successful only if it is important enough to become a part of your daily routine.

Determining Conditioning Needs

The first step in designing a total body conditioning program is that of selecting exercises which will meet your individual needs. Perhaps the importance of making wise exercise choices is best illustrated by looking at the leotard-clad gymnasts or competitive swimmers who perform in the Olympics. You see strong, supple, well-proportioned bodies performing with a beauty and grace that you appreciate. Bulky, protruding "amazon" type muscles are conspicuously absent among these performers. Appropriate conditioning builds strong bodies, yet enhances a woman's femininity and emphasizes a man's masculinity. This is what a sound conditioning program should and will accomplish.

Because inherited, physical characteristics, environmental influences, and daily living routines are so diverse, individual body conditioning needs are as different as personalities. You inherited a particular skeletal framework which no amount of exercise will alter. You also inherited a kind of predisposition to accumulate fatty body tissue. But substantially the shape you develop on your bony structure is left squarely up to you. For example, through disuse your muscles become flaccid whereas with appropriate physical conditioning they will be firm. Likewise, as a result of minimal physical activity you accumulate bulky, unsightly, cumbersome fat deposits while suitable physical activity and conditioning helps you avoid these fat deposits.

In addition, a myriad of environmental factors will affect your physique. Generally speaking, American homes are filled with labor-saving devices and the same is true of schools, offices, farms, and the like. Such conveniences obviously tend to minimize vigorous use of the body while encouraging a sedentary existence.

Through research, exercise physiologists have identified three basic conditioning needs which are necessary for everyone irrespective of constitutional body type, environs, and work routines. A basic conditioning program should include exercises designed to:

1. Develop muscle strength and endurance in all major muscle groups of the body; the neck, chest, upper arm and shoulder girdle, abdomen and lower back, hips, legs, and feet.
2. Increase flexibility in the major body joints; the spine, shoulders, hips, knees, ankles, and feet.
3. Improve the efficiency of the heart, lungs, and blood vessels by increasing circulorespiratory endurance.

Your personal concern should be to condition your body to the point where you can perform the work tasks required of you and the recreational activities you choose without becoming fatigued in the process. That is to say, if you are a student you should be able to attend classes, study, play, and work at a job during a normal day and still have an energy reserve. Further, you should wake up each morning rested and relaxed, with a body that is prepared to complete the activities of the day.

Remember, your potential for achieving the goals of your day will have to be enhanced by your muscle strength and circulorespiratory endurance or limited by your muscle weakness and circulorespiratory inefficiency.

Implementing the Conditioning Program

You may design an excellent conditioning program but unless you perform each of the exercises included in it accurately and adequately you will not realize the desired conditioning gains. As you prepare to design your exercise program the following suggestions should be helpful:

1. Follow carefully the description given for the performance of each exercise. Every exercise is designed for a specific purpose and when you change it (either intentionally or unintentionally) you run the risk of spending effort and time doing exercises which will not lead to achievement of the intended purposes. It is also possible that changing an exercise may result in placing body joints in a position which may actually be injurious to the muscle tissue or the joint.
2. Avoid selecting exercises which will accentuate a postural deviation that you are trying to improve or eliminate.
3. When choosing exercises from books and other sources be certain that the authors are professionally qualified people. Be discerning when selecting exercises from current home-making and fashion magazines.

Maintaining a High Level of Physical Condition

Having achieved a level of total body conditioning adequate for your needs, your final concern will be with maintaining that status for a lifetime. You don't gain a well-conditioned body by a process of osmosis. Neither will you maintain it by desire alone. It is important to understand that, once established, the well-conditioned appearance and feeling of your body can be maintained largely through participation in socially enjoyable and physically stimulating sports activities. The selection of these recreational activities will be determined by your personal preferences. Decide what sports you enjoy or think you would enjoy and pursue them regularly. Then plan a brief supplementary program keeping the following in mind:

1. Determine what, if any, further special conditioning you need to improve your readiness for participation in the sports or activities selected.
2. Be sure to plan for the strength, flexibility, and circulo-respiratory needs that will not be met through your recreational activities.
3. Include exercises designed to improve postural alignment.

At this point you might reasonably ask, "Is it worth the effort?" Ultimately only you can decide. The benefits are very real. It is possible to observe the vigor, spirit, drive, and enthusiasm for living that is a continuing characteristic of the "physically fit" individual. One can point to the brisk step, graceful movements, and poised carriage and feel deep appreciation for the model. Significant, too, are the values which have been identified by the medical profession—values which relate to delaying the physical appearance of aging and to increasing life expectancy, to one's self-image, and to one's ability to resist disease and illness or avoid unnecessary injury.

In the final analysis, many of the benefits of a life conditioning program are of an intrinsic nature and their worth will never be completely realized until the state of physical conditioning necessary to experience them is achieved. Where these indefinable qualities are concerned, self-realization will come only through self-experience. Most of you recognize and appreciate a well-conditioned body when you see it and when you see such a person you realize somehow that the appearance, behaviors, and characteristics your eyes behold are a visible manifestation of an inner vitality and energy reserve which must exist. You don't adequately measure, or indeed describe, such values as these until you have experienced them. This enviable state of optimal physical condition does exist for some people and it can exist for you. Perhaps herein lies your challenge.

Summary of Basic Concepts

1. Your dynamic conditioning program should be highly individualized and therefore specialized.
2. The success of a conditioning program ultimately rests with your conscientious persistence.
3. You have achieved a state of adequate conditioning for daily living when you can perform your required work tasks and participate in recreational activities without becoming fatigued.
4. It is absolutely essential to perform selected exercises correctly.
5. Maintenance of an optimal level of conditioning can be accomplished largely through regular participation in sports activities supplemented by selected exercises.

Chapter 2

THE DYNAMIC CONDITIONING PROGRAM

Muscle Strength and Endurance

In American society it seems quite possible that girls and women associate strength with the physical force and power which they most often see demonstrated in their male counterparts. Then, too, perhaps "strength" is such an ordinary word that we fail to consider its meaning with reference to the role it plays in our personal, everyday living. In either case, it seems necessary to evaluate your own strength and determine whether or not the amount you possess actually enables you to do what you desire as well as what your responsibilities require. Do you have the strength you need to easily lift a box of heavy household items and place it on a shelf? Does your present level of strength enhance or restrict the effectiveness of your tennis stroke or the way you control your bowling ball? The strength and endurance capacity of your muscles plays a vital role in the effective and successful performance of these and countless other daily living activities.

One of the primary purposes of your conditioning program will be to increase the working effectiveness of your muscles. Fortunately, all normal muscles possess some degree of strength. This is because some muscular fibers are constantly stimulated by nerve impulses so that some tension (tone) is always present in muscle. But muscles which are exercised minimally tend to be flaccid; they have poor tone; they are "lazy" muscles. When you improve muscle tone and develop *muscle strength,* you increase the amount of force muscles can exert or the amount of work they can perform.

Muscles are extremely versatile body tissues which have the ability to shorten (contract) and return to their original length (relax). In addition, they have the capacity to become tense or tight without appreciably changing their length. It is the combination of these characteristics plus their strategic points of attachment to bones which makes it possible for you to work, to play, even to move.

7

As you extend the ability of your muscles to work strenuously for progressively longer periods of time you are developing *muscle endurance.* As you increase muscle strength you also increase muscle endurance. When you lift a heavy load correctly you are demonstrating the strength of your legs, upper arms, and shoulder muscles. You test the endurance of these muscles by noting either how far the load can be carried or how many times the lift can be repeated, without rest, before fatigue makes it necessary to stop.

In order to increase the strength of muscles it is necessary to tax them. To develop strength you will need to gradually increase the amount of work your muscles are required to do in the exercises you select. You will work your muscles to the point of literally fatiguing them. This is the only way you can improve strength, and the method has been designated as the *overload principle.*

Two typical methods of developing strength which utilize the overload principle are known as *isotonic* and *isometric* exercise. Isotonic exercise involves moving the body (or limbs) through a given range of motion by contracting and relaxing certain muscles. The resistance the muscles are working against is continually overcome. In isometric exercise the muscles used develop tension as a position is assumed, held, and then released. The muscles work against resistance which will not be overcome. These two types of exercising can be illustrated by analyzing two versions of a modified push-up. The push-up demonstrated in Figure 1 is an isotonic exercise. The body is repeatedly moved through the prescribed range of movement by being alternately raised and lowered. Figure 2 shows an isometric push-up. The body is partially lowered and then this position is held for a specified time.

You should always include isotonic exercises in a conditioning program. Isometric exercises are suggested as a supplement because

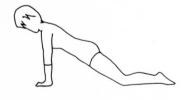

Figure 1   Figure 2

they do not contribute appreciably to improved circulorespiratory endurance and they contribute nothing to the development of flexibility. As a matter of fact, when used exclusively, isometrics are undesirable because they develop strength only at the angle of contraction held and tend to decrease flexibility.

Because strength-developing exercises make a strenuous demand on muscles, you should expect to experience some feelings of discomfort while performing them. As you continue to perform the exercise this discomfort, which is slight at first, gradually increases. But when you complete the exercise and release the tension on the muscle, the discomfort promptly ceases. It is important to understand that this feeling in the working muscles is both natural and necessary in the strength-developing process. If you fail to experience this physical discomfort you are not making the muscles work hard enough.

There is a second type of discomfort which is associated with strength exercises. Within a day or two after you have exercised muscles which have not been accustomed to doing hard work, you may feel some stiffness and soreness. This happens because during exercise waste products build up in the muscles faster than they can be removed. You will discover that the soreness disappears most readily if you continue your regular exercise and activity routine, and it will not ordinarily recur as long as you follow a progressive daily conditioning program.

The condition of your muscles has a great deal to do with your overall appearance. Toned muscles definitely improve body contours. Flaccid muscles make it extremely difficult, if not impossible, to maintain an attractive posture. Lazy muscles tire easily and are frequently the cause of mid-afternoon or early-evening fatigue, fatigue that is unwelcome because it arrives before studies are completed or before the party begins. Sluggish muscles respond slowly and make it difficult to manipulate your body with the control needed on the tennis courts or the ski slopes. There is no question about it—it takes real determination and effort to attain a desirable level of total body strength. But those who will work to attain it should know that maintaining optimum strength requires notably less effort while yielding the same valuable benefits. Hopefully, reflecting on the merits of possessing adequate strength will motivate you to improve yours.

Circulorespiratory Endurance

In this phase of your conditioning program your heart and lungs combine their efforts in a most intricate manner in order to improve what is known as your circulorespiratory endurance. This quality identifies the ability of your circulorespiratory system to transport oxygen and nutrients to muscles. Ultimately the oxygen serves as a catalyst for the chemical reactions of muscular contraction. When you stop to realize that the body cannot store oxygen as it does food, you will recognize the tremendous importance of an efficient circulorespiratory system.

Working together, your heart and lungs carry oxygen and nutrients to, and remove carbon dioxide from, the working muscles. It is this process that furnishes the muscles with the energy they need to perform work. Without question your heart is the most amazing muscle in your body. It has been described as being about the size of a man's hand and is said to weigh less than a pound. Yet the heart beats for a lifetime, faithfully pumping blood throughout the human body. By conditioning your heart and blood vessels (circulatory system) you increase the amount of blood your heart pumps with each beat. This is known as the stroke volume of the heart. It is important to realize that because the heart is a muscle it must be conditioned in much the same manner as any muscle. It will become stronger and larger and will operate more efficiently when properly conditioned. In other words, the heart can be trained to work more effectively. Just as any normal body muscle will benefit positively from exercise, so too will your heart muscle. But the converse is also true. The heart, as any muscle, will become weakened as a result of inadequate or inappropriate use. The strong heart will perform with greater efficiency than the weak heart in several important ways: it will pump more blood with each beat; it will not beat as often (the heart "rests" between beats); and it will return to its normal resting state sooner following strenuous exertion.

It is natural for your heart to beat noticeably faster during activity. As you begin your conditioning program the increased rate of your heartbeat may give you one index of how hard you are working. Eventually, as your conditioning level improves, you will notice that both your resting and your exercising heartbeats (rates) are slower than they were before you started your conditioning program. This means that your heart is pumping more blood with each beat; consequently, it doesn't need to beat as often. Nevertheless, vigorous activity will speed up the heartbeat and it should not be surprising if, during vigorous activity, your heartbeat increases as much as two and one-half times its normal resting rate. The heart of the physically unfit person works much harder to accomplish the same amount of work than does the heart of the person who has attained a high level of fitness. In other words, the heart of the physically well-conditioned individual increases its stroke volume much more readily than does that of the unconditioned individual. Furthermore, the pulse rate of the conditioned person will return to normal more quickly after the exercise has stopped.

The lungs also perform a vital function in the improvement of your circulorespiratory endurance. During prolonged activity your muscle tissues require additional amounts of oxygen, above and beyond that needed when you are relatively inactive. By developing the capacity of your lungs and respiratory system you can increase the amount of oxygen exchanged during each breath. This is known as the tidal volume of your lungs. Since the lungs do not store oxygen it is only by increasing their vital capacity that the lungs can furnish the amount of oxygen needed by the muscles if vigorous activity is to be sustained. It is also normal for your respiratory rate to increase during activity. You breathe faster. When you first begin the endurance exercises notice that you breathe heavily and will possibly feel quite breathless. After several weeks of faithful exercise, during which you "push" yourself, you will notice that you are not breathless in spite of the fact that you are exercising much harder than you were in the beginning. This is an indication that your circulorespiratory endurance is improving.

Clearly, the value of increasing circulorespiratory endurance has to be regarded as extremely significant when you are dealing with such vital and priceless organs as your heart and lungs. The amount of research and skill currently being directed toward establishing vital organ banks and perfecting organ transplants should serve as a constant reminder of the importance of their conservation.

Flexibility

The graceful, flowing movement observed in the well-conditioned individual is largely a function of flexibility. Hence, the degree of joint flexibility you possess will be a primary determinant of the quality of your body movements. Flexibility is the term used to describe the range of motion in your body joints. This range may be too great as well as too limited, and you need to consider the problems connected with both extremes.

Your capacity to increase flexibility is determined by heredity and environment. Neither the length of bones nor the joint structure can be altered appreciably because they are inherited. There are, however, other factors influencing flexibility over which you have decided control, and it is with these that we are primarily concerned. For example, fat deposits and bulky muscles around a joint will decrease the range of motion in that joint. Through correct diet and exercise you can usually prevent or eliminate both of these problems. For most of us joint flexibility depends upon the degree of muscular strength and elasticity we possess. These qualities are also within individual control.

A brief explanation of the structure and function of the joints should help to clarify the vital role muscles play in increasing flexibility. Joints are formed when two bones come together. Ligaments and muscles bind the joint which is formed when the two bones meet. Thus, the stability of the joint is largely determined by the condition of these ligaments and muscles.

Ligaments are largely tough, nonelastic type fibers which join the two bones and help to hold them in correct alignment. The small percentage of elastic fibers that are found in the ligaments provide a margin of safety when the range of movement in the joint borders on the extreme as a result of too much pressure or pull being placed on the joint. When sufficient force is applied, ligaments may be stretched or torn. Unfortunately once a ligament is stretched it remains stretched. As a result, its contribution to the stability of the joint will always be considerably reduced. In this latter situation optimal muscle development is imperative for the protection of the joint.

Muscles are elastic fibers which cross the joints and also attach to both bones. It is their elastic quality that makes it normal for muscles to both contract (shorten) and relax (lengthen). Muscles are arranged in pairs and usually cross the joint on opposite sides. It is this pairing of muscles which makes movement in a joint possible because when one of the muscles contracts the opposing muscle automatically relaxes. When sufficient force is applied against it a given muscle may be stretched beyond its normal resting length. The best way to safely stretch a muscle, thereby increasing its elasticity, is to tighten the muscle which opposes it.

To develop adequate flexibility you will need to do exercises which require the muscles surrounding the joint to both contract and relax. To say it another way, muscular strengthening exercises which consistently sustain the normal range of motion in joints will also maintain the elasticity of the muscles surrounding the joint. It is important to note the kinds of movements required of your body in the performance of daily work tasks and other habitual activities before you select flexibility exercises for your conditioning program. Some activities require either more or less flexibility in a given joint or joints than others. For example, the dancer, the swimmer, and the gymnast seek more than normal flexibility, while average amounts are adequate for the bowler or golfer. Such specialized needs should also be taken into consideration in your conditioning program design.

When performing flexibility exercises it is important to stretch the muscles progressively, slowly, smoothly, and cautiously. Successive performances should stretch and hold the muscle slightly beyond its existing comfortable length. You should feel the "pull" on the muscle during sustained stretching movements. There are several "do nots" which must be carefully observed. Do not make unreasonable stretching demands on the muscles. Avoid exercises which call for quick, jerky, bouncing type movements. Do not add weights to increase the pull on the muscle. Approach the task of developing flexibility intelligently. Work gradually and patiently, for it takes time to increase flexibility.

Relaxation

Have you had the experience of lying in bed wide awake even though you were very tired and wanted to sleep? Have you ever felt as though you were "tied in knots" while waiting to give a speech or for the professor to distribute the final course examination? Whether we realize it or not, most of us experience this type of tension because our body responds to mental, social, and emotional tension with physical (muscular) tension.

The variety of stresses that daily living responsibilities impose on all of us make it necessary that we learn how to release unnecessary muscle tension. This unnecessary tension interferes with coordinated performance, results in loss of efficiency, and hastens the onset of both physical and mental fatigue. In the human body, relaxation is possible because we can learn to release tension in muscles. We relax when we consciously release unnecessary, hence undesirable, tension. But while it is possible, it is not always easy to release tension. For many people the release of unwanted muscle tension is a deliberate learning process which requires thoughtful concentration.

The best approach to the problem of excessive tension is to remove the cause, but realistically this is not always possible. A second approach may be found in pursuing recreational activities that are enjoyable and relaxing because they divert one's attention from the tension causers. Relaxation through recreation should be incorporated into every individual's living routine. A third approach involves increasing one's ability to feel muscle tension when it is present, to consciously and purposefully release it and feel the reduction of tension. The exercises in this text are designed to utilize this last approach. These methods emphasize the need for thoughtful concentration on the feeling of relaxed or "loose" muscles. Many times the concentration diverts one's attention from a tension-producing situation, thereby making a significant contribution to the relaxation effort. Try to perform relaxation exercises in warm, pleasant, quiet surroundings. While it is important that you be comfortable, be sure that the surface on which you are exercising offers firm support for your body. For some people soft, soothing music will be conducive to relaxation while for others it distracts from concentration. The number of repetitions of the exercise or the time devoted to it must be individually determined. See how long it takes before you feel relaxed. You seek suppleness, looseness, and a serene, composed feeling. Since increasing one's capacity to relax appears to be a universal human need, begin experimenting with these methods. Learning to relax will be beneficial now and will help to prepare you for the inevitable anxieties and events which are known to take a tremendous toll in the mental and physical well-being of our society.

Remember that relaxation is a learned skill. It requires deliberate concentration and practice. The ability to relax is not learned in a day but once you possess it you may achieve it any day.

Summary of Basic Concepts

1. Muscle strength refers to the amount of force a muscle can exert or the amount of work it can perform.
2. Muscular endurance is the capacity of a muscle to exert force over an extended time period without fatigue.
3. Muscular strength is increased when a muscle is made to work against a progressively increased resistance.
4. Circulorespiratory endurance is the ability of the heart and lungs to supply oxygen to muscles over an extended time period or under conditions of stress.
5. The heart is a muscle and will therefore benefit positively from exercise.
6. It is normal for the heart and respiratory rate to increase during vigorous activity.
7. Flexibility, or the range of motion in joints, is the physical capacity which permits graceful, flowing movement.
8. Muscles are arranged in pairs; the elasticity of one muscle is directly related to the strength of its opposing muscle.
9. Flexibility can be maintained or increased by exercises which slowly and progressively stretch a muscle beyond its resting length.
10. Stress-producing situations are always accompanied by muscular tension which contributes to fatigue.
11. Participation in recreational activities and conscious relaxation are two recommended techniques for tension reduction.

Chapter 3

THE SPECIFIC CONDITIONING PROGRAM

RELATED PHYSICAL CONCERNS

Mobility

Your mobility—your readiness to move and the ease with which you move—will be considerably enhanced when your muscles are strong and your flexibility is optimal. Some qualities of movement so readily observed in others are difficult to define. The ability to move with power yet with dexterity is apparent as you watch a halfback weave his way through an opponent's defensive line. The sprinter leaving the starting blocks demonstrates an action which is both explosive and fluid. The gymnast is constantly making strong movements while maintaining balance and suppleness of body and limb.

The freedom to move gracefully is learned, but the learning is based on body condition. Make no mistake, the individual who displays grace in form and action has made the effort necessary to develop optimum strength, endurance, and flexibility without which beautiful movement is impossible.

Weight Management

In a modern society where mechanized conveniences and excessive eating seem to be a way of life, where spectator sports are booming and work tasks requiring vigorous exertion have virtually vanished into obscurity, it is logical that overweight and obesity prevail. This is the condition evidenced in America today. It exists because it is typical for Americans to eat too much and exercise too little.

When discussing the problems associated with weight control, some authorities use the words overweight and obesity interchangeably. Others make a distinction regarding the proportion of body fat

17

in relationship to muscle. They define overweight as being weight in excess of "normal" and obesity as fat in excess of "normal." Still others indicate that an overweight individual is ten pounds or more over the "ideal" weight and the obese individual is twenty pounds or more over the "ideal" weight. The problem with these definitions comes in determining what the "normal" or "ideal" weight for any given individual should be. Nutrition experts do not agree on these criteria and are constantly seeking better means for determining what constitutes "normal" or "ideal" weight. It seems obvious that, whatever definition one uses, overweight and/or obese persons carry a surplus of fatty tissue.

When the subject of individual weight problems is discussed, several questions are among the first to be raised. Isn't most excessive weight primarily a problem of metabolism rate? Some of us are large-boned, so won't we naturally weigh more than the smaller-boned person? Isn't it usually glandular problems that cause obesity?

The diet, nutrition, and weight management authorities tell us that the weight of bones is almost identical in persons of a given height. They warn us that too many people lay the cause of their obesity at the basal metabolism doorstep. And, with tongue in cheek, they suggest that most professed glandular problems are, in reality, "salivary" gland problems. It is true that genetic factors may predispose an individual to obesity, but usually a person becomes overweight as a result of consuming more calories than the body uses. The experts urge us to remember that the primary concern, for most of us, is fat; not bone structure, not genetic factors, and not glandular disturbances.

Recent research identifies two factors which are commonly related to obesity: heredity and a low level of activity. It has been determined that at low levels of activity (referred to as the sedentary range) the weight control mechanisms of the human body do not function properly. It has been well established that an affluent society is highly conducive to sedentary living; hence too many Americans are overweight or obese. Someone has said that *Homo sapiens* has become *Homo sedentarius.* And there are two evolutionary stages still open to the human species: *Homo sportius* and *Homo obesus.*

There are several methods you may use to determine whether or not your weight and its distribution are appropriate for you. You may test for overweight by standing in a leotard in front of a mirror. What do you see? Like poor posture, your fat shows. Or take the "pinch test" by grasping the skin and fat just above your waist between your thumb and forefinger. You should be able to pinch no more than one inch (one-half inch would be ideal). Make the same test on your buttocks, your abdomen, and at the back of your upper arm. You may want to check your weight against the desirable weight suggested on the weight chart. The weight chart used does not

	HEIGHT (with shoes on) 2-inch heels		SMALL	MEDIUM	LARGE
	Feet	Inches	FRAME	FRAME	FRAME
	4	10	92– 98	96–107	104–119
Women	4	11	94–101	98–110	106–122
of Ages 25	5	0	96–104	101–113	109–125
and Over	5	1	99–107	104–116	112–128
	5	2	102–110	107–119	115–131
	5	3	105–113	110–122	118–134
	5	4	108–116	113–126	121–138
	5	5	111–119	116–130	125–142
	5	6	114–123	120–135	129–146
	5	7	118–127	124–139	133–150
	5	8	122–131	128–143	137–154
	5	9	126–135	132–147	141–158
	5	10	130–140	136–151	145–163
	5	11	134–144	140–155	149–168
	6	0	138–148	144–159	153–173

Metropolitan Life Weight Chart
Courtesy of the Metropolitan Life Insurance Company

suggest age range categories because that type of guide just seems to reflect the fact that Americans get fatter as they get older. The weights given on the chart here are for women wearing indoor clothing and shoes with a two-inch heel. If you usually weigh on a bathroom scale wearing nothing but a towel, subtract two to four pounds. Be sure to use the same scale and take your weight at the same time each day. Scales will vary. Also, you are likely to weigh less in the morning than in the afternoon. If it is important to you to obtain a more specific weight measurement it is possible to approximate your frame classification by measuring the wrist above the bone on your nondominant hand. The large frame measurement will be 6-1/4 to 6-3/4 inches; medium will be 5-1/2 to 6-1/8 inches; and a small frame will be 4-1/2 to 5-1/8 inches. These should be regarded as general guidelines. Because they are guidelines they may not apply specifically to you. The "chart" weight suggested for you may seem too heavy or too light. It might make you feel like a blimp or it could trim you down to a shadow. If your actual weight falls slightly outside the range recommended for one of your size and build, yet you feel well and you know you look attractive, it may be best for you to simply concern yourself with maintaining your present weight and keeping your muscles toned. Some people who like to take "before" and "after" girth measurements do not understand how their measurements can decrease without weight loss. The explanation is that muscle weighs more than fat; hence, it is quite possible for you to lose inches without losing pounds. In this situation the significant factor is the improvement in appearance which should be most apparent in the fit of your clothes and the reflection in your mirror.

These methods can be most useful in helping you to discover problems of underweight and/or overweight. However, failure to fall into one of these two categories does not exclude you from being concerned about weight control. Do you like rich foods? Do you eat heartily? Do you tend to shun physical exercise? Are you over twenty? If your answer to any one of these questions is "yes," you need to understand the basic principles of weight management.

Weight control is based on a simple concept: the food and beverages we consume contain calories (units of energy). The body burns these calories in activity. The most common cause of excessive weight is easily pinpointed when we realize that any calories which are not used are stored in the body as fat. Hence, if your problem is one of overweight you will need to exercise more and eat less. If you are underweight, you need to consume more calories than your body uses until you reach a desirable weight. If your weight is desirable, you can maintain it by making certain that your caloric intake equals your energy output.

In cases of severe overweight or underweight it is best to consult your physician and follow his recommendations with respect to both diet and exercise. Medical authorities are expressing deep concern about the health problems caused by overweight. Some of their concerns relate to research which indicates that overweight shortens life expectancy, inhibits recovery from heart attacks, complicates surgical procedures, increases the incidence of chronic and degenerative disease, and causes undesirable and unnecessary strains on the weight-bearing joints of the body.

Most Americans need a reeducation in diet that includes a knowledge of the caloric content of foods and the caloric values of exercise. Where eating is concerned, indiscriminate dieting or wholesale overindulgence is dangerous. With respect to curbing caloric intake, remember the body has basic nutritional needs in order to function properly, so a decreased intake must always maintain a proportionate nutritional balance. If you want to lose more than two pounds per week or more than a total of ten pounds you should seek medical advice.

Many foods provide both calories and essential nutrients (vitamins, minerals, proteins) needed to build the body and keep it in good working condition. Other foods high in fat or carbohydrates provide little besides energy. The calories from these foods are sometimes called "empty" calories. Stay with the recommended "basic four" food groups: milk, meat, vegetables-fruits, and bread-cereal. Eat three light meals daily. Eat slowly and load up on fillers; carrots, celery, consommes, and most fresh fruits. Get a calorie counter book and check your diet carefully with it. If you need a snack, use part of your regular caloric allotment. There is considerable evidence that concentrating the food intake into one or two large meals results in a greater tendency toward obesity. There is also evidence that the obese tend to eat heavily in the evening.

Opinions regarding the role that exercise plays in weight management have fluctuated from "very little" to "very important." Recent research studies clearly indicate that increasing physical exercise is now considered at least as important as decreasing food consumption. Physicians are currently pointing to the lack of physical activity as a significant cause of "creeping overweight." This term refers to a gradual increase in weight which comes about slowly over a period of several years. After the age of twenty, there is a gradual reduction in the metabolic rate, so extra poundage can creep on even if the caloric output and intake remain constant. If you become less active, the rate of weight increase can be faster. You will not be troubled with creeping overweight if you make certain that your physical activity is sufficient to use the few excess calories you might otherwise accumulate each day. How well you maintain this balance between diet and exercise will play a major role in determining your weight constancy and your appearance.

There seem to be two particularly misleading notions held by some people with respect to exercise and weight control. One of these misconceptions says that exercise automatically increases one's appetite to the point where the calories expended through exercise are constantly replaced because one eats more. Experimental evidence indicates two things: the first is that, within a moderate range of activity, exercise need not stimulate the appetite appreciably and, second, exercise has a regulating effect on the appetite. Further, when you overwork physically you tend to lose your appetite. A second fallacy suggests that one needs to devote a great deal of time and effort to exercise in order to lose weight. It is true that you must burn a substantial number of calories to lose a pound of stored fat, but you don't have to do this in a single effort. Accumulatively you can "spend" a great number of calories when you engage in regular activity over an extended period of time. it has been demonstrated that thirty minutes of appropriate exercise each day for one year can result in a weight loss of over twenty-five pounds.

Many people seem to be looking for a quick and easy way to shed unwanted pounds. Consequently, there is a big market for appetite depressants, weight control aids, diet foods, fad and crash diets, and machines of the vibrating and rolling variety. If there is an easy, fast, yet safe way to lose excessive weight, that method is yet to be discovered. Crash diets involving rapid weight losses are dangerous because they do not give the body the time it needs to adjust to the changes in body tissue. Dehydration results in a loss of fluid which the body needs to facilitate the elimination of body wastes. In both cases the weight loss is only temporary since the appetite is not changed. Dietetic foods must be carefully selected. The sugar content in dietetic foods is low, but the fat content is not always correspondingly low.

Machines are often expensive gimmicks which are of little value because you cannot squeeze or vibrate calories out of the body. Many diet aids have addictive properties. Drugs and pills are costly and when used extensively are a tremendous waste of money. In addition the effect of drugs will be gradually lost over a period of time. Failure to get enough sleep, a seemingly chronic condition of the college student, may produce a temporary weight loss. You should recognize that this is an undesirable approach to weight control because it reduces the general efficiency of the body and because it can contribute to a high susceptibility to disease.

Most of us need to accept the fact that we cannot eat everything we like nor as much as we like. It is as simple as that. There is no substitute for willpower and vigorous physical activity. It has been suggested that we regard weight management as a "living" insurance which costs persistent determination and approximately two pounds of sweat per week.

Menstruation and Dysmenorrhea

The menstrual cycle is a normal and natural physiological function which is indicative of the onset of puberty and usually first occurs between the ages of twelve and thirteen. Because of individual differences some girls will experience menarche earlier, while for a few it will begin later. Ordinarily the cycle recurs every twenty-eight to thirty days; however, irregularity is not uncommon during the first few months. Such inconstancies may be caused by circumstances such as environmental changes, unexpected emotional upsets, extreme nervous tension, and certain types of illnesses.

Many women experience a change in body temperature and some pain, or dysmenorrhea, just prior to and during the first day or two of each menstrual cycle. This discomfort is usually as major or minor as you choose to make it. Some women tend to indulge themselves by remaining in bed, avoiding physical exercise or consuming quantities of pain relievers. Medical authorities suggest that relatively few cases (approximately 25 per cent) of cramps, nausea, head and backaches are organic in origin. Gynecologists appear to agree that women who experience a relatively normal menstrual cycle will benefit from regular mild to vigorous exercise during menstruation. Not infrequently the woman who is very inactive or the woman whose diet is not well balanced experiences unnecessary physical discomfort. This is true because regular exercise promotes blood circulation and a balanced diet helps to avert constipation, thus tending to alleviate some of the causes of pain and cramps. In addition, it has been hypothesized that emotional stresses and excessive muscle tension which cause undue pressure on certain local nerves may contribute to physical discomfort. Poorly balanced posture has also been suggested as a condition which adds to lower back discomfort during menstruation; however, this theory does not appear to have been substantiated by research.

In cases of such obvious irregularities as prolonged fluctuations in the menstrual cycle, severe lower abdominal and back pain, hemorrhaging or hypertension, it would be most advisable to consult with a physician to determine whether specific exercises should be prescribed or whether exercise is entirely contraindicated.

Physicians who have studied the problems associated with menstrual discomfort have designed and recommended some specific exercises, which, if performed regularly, will often prevent dysmenorrhea. The exercises suggested for dysmenorrhea in this text are representative of those which often eliminate or relieve menstrual pain. In addition, it is recommended that the exercises designed to develop abdominal strength are also valuable in this regard.

CONDITIONING FOR SPORT SKILLS

We have been called a nation of spectators and it is true that too many of us let our own machinery rust while we watch others lubricate theirs. As "watchers" we tend to get our "kicks" vicariously while the performer's benefits are obtained first-hand. The adult who during childhood and adolescence has been encouraged to learn skills and participate in a variety of sports, games, and other forms of physical exercise is indeed fortunate. Such a person is likely to have developed a continuing interest in selected activities to the extent that they become lifetime pursuits. Those whose participation has been relatively limited will find it necessary to explore activities and identify those on which they wish to concentrate. Selecting several activities is most acceptable. It seems important to realize that you tend to continually involve yourself in a sport, game, aquatic, or dance activity when your performance is reasonably proficient.

Participating actively in sports and recreational activities is an enjoyable means of maintaining a well-conditioned body. As has been suggested previously, you retain only the range of motion, strength, and endurance that you regularly use. Select sports that you like and participate in them on a regular basis. Choose activities that you can enjoy with your family and friends for the rest of your life. There is considerable food for thought in the phrase which suggests "the family that plays together stays together." And certainly one's capacity to play a respectable game of golf or tennis may be a social or business asset as well as a means of physical conditioning. It is also a fact that a person who has been in the habit of participating regularly in active sports will find it easier to adjust to retirement than one who does so only occasionally.

We often do skilled performers an injustice when we attribute their skill to a natural ability. Learning sport skills, some of which are quite complicated, will take desire, time, persistence, good instruction, accurate practice, and appropriate conditioning. One does not become skilled in a few short weeks. Teachers of beginning sport skills are continually faced with students unable to perform the most basic skills successfully because of poor physical conditioning. Consider carefully your present physical condition and the level of conditioning needed to take on the challenges of learning a new skill. As was suggested in Chapter 1, your "physical readiness" to learn is a critical factor and you may be certain that your learning will be facilitated if your body is in optimal condition before your instruction begins.

INDIVIDUAL SPORTS

Archery

Archery is basically a sport of accuracy and the ability to adjust to shooting at varied distances. There are several sources of error which can impair accuracy from any given distance. Most of these are related to inadequate muscle strength, muscle endurance, or relaxation factors.

Skilled performance in archery will require better-than-average strength of arms, shoulder, and upper back muscles. In addition, the archer needs thigh and trunk strength sufficient to assume and maintain a fixed, stable, erect alignment throughout the draw, aim, and release of the arrow. It is customary to match the strength of the bow to the relative strength of the archer. But to become a skilled woman target archer you should be able to easily draw a twenty-six to twenty-eight pound bow. You must be able then, to draw against a twenty-six pound resistance and perform the action smoothly. To do so, the muscles in your arms, shoulders, and upper back must remain contracted, holding these parts of the body virtually motionless until the arrow has left the bow. Ability to hold this fixed position repeatedly demands a high level of muscle strength and endurance. The leg strength developed in your general conditioning program should be sufficient for the stability demands made on the archer in target shooting.

The general conditioning program should also be adequate for the range of motion in body joints as well as the circulorespiratory endurance required for skilled archery performance.

The stance of the archer should be erect, stable, and firm. It should also be a stance which is free of unnecessary muscle tension. Secondly, the thumb and fingers of your bow hand should simply encircle the bow. They should not grip it tightly. As the string is drawn, the pressure of the bow exerted against your hand will hold the bow in place. Finally, improper release of the arrow is an error commonly experienced by beginning archers. The arrow is released by simply relaxing your fingers, only your fingers. The ability to consciously relax specific muscle groups will be a definite asset to you in perfecting your archery skills.

Badminton

Badminton can be played and enjoyed as a family activity or a strenuous, highly competitive tournament game.

To play a better-than-average game in either type of play the wrist "snap" is such a critical action that special attention should be given to the development of good wrist strength and flexibility. The light racket used in badminton makes your wrist snap the most significant single contributor to the speed of the shuttlecock in flight. Strong, well-toned leg muscles will facilitate your efforts to make the quick stops, starts, and changes of direction required in good badminton play. Since underhand return shots are principally defensive shots the best return shot is an overhand stroke. To be in a position of "readiness" to return an opponent's shot quickly, your racket should be held well up in front of the body. Your general conditioning program should provide you with the strength which will enable you to assume this position repeatedly throughout the game. If you find that you are unable to hold the racket high while waiting for the opponent's return you should work to increase your upper arm and shoulder strength to the point where you can.

The greater the flexibility in the wrist joint, the more effective will be the wrist action. Increase the range of motion in your wrist joint and you will increase the arc through which the racket can move, thereby increasing the force which can be imparted to the shuttle. Your general conditioning program should provide the flexibility needed in other body joints.

Whether you have been involved in family games or in tournaments, a high level of circulorespiratory endurance will improve your game. As with tennis, a strenuous game of badminton calls for considerable movement, sudden movement, fast movement, fatiguing movement. An average level of circulorespiratory endurance is likely to impose limitations on your game, particularly when you are opposing a player whose skill matches yours.

As has been suggested, replacing muscle tension with muscle relaxation at strategic times will result in decreased energy expenditure, more fluid movements, and more effective stroke execution. Ultimately, then, your ability to relax muscles at will makes a significant contribution to the caliber of game you play.

Bowling

Successful bowling demands a combination of speed and accuracy. The bowler must learn to transfer the momentum generated in the approach to the ball and, at the same time, be accurate enough to hit a three-quarter inch spot which is sixteen feet from the foul line.

Generally, heavy balls produce greater pinfall than light ones. It is desirable, therefore, for you to roll a fourteen to sixteen pound ball. To control a heavy ball and still have adequate speed you will need a substantial level of strength in the hand, wrist, arm, and shoulder. Accuracy will be achieved only when the ball is released from a consistent, stable body position. This stability is dependent upon a high degree of leg strength, since the leg opposite the bowling arm must overcome the forward momentum of your body and balance against the force of the moving weight of the ball.

Some flexibility is needed in your shoulder girdle to facilitate an adequately high backswing. However, most beginners find that lack of strength, rather than lack of flexibility, is the inhibiting factor.

Circulorespiratory endurance is not a critical component of bowling achievement because the bowler is not called upon for uninterrupted performance. The very fact that there is a waiting period while the ball is returned provides you with an automatic rest period.

As in most skilled movement patterns, relaxation plays a vital role. The steps in the approach should be graceful, smooth, and "easy," while the armswing is natural and fluid. The bowler must learn to relax sufficiently to permit the weight of the ball to determine the path of the swing, while maintaining enough muscular tension to impart the necessary force. Conscious relaxation may be helpful in learning to achieve this alternate action between relaxation and tension.

Contemporary Dance

The relationship between conditioning and successful performance in contemporary dance is, at best, enigmatic. On the one hand a high level of conditioning can only serve to facilitate performance but on the other hand a high level of conditioning is not an absolute prerequisite of a satisfying dance experience. The explanation for this ambiguous relationship rests with the function of creativity and self-motivation in this activity.

The ultimate goal of "the dance" is self-expression through movement. If you have a consuming desire to express an idea you can sometimes overcome, or at least compensate for, your physical inadequacies and thus achieve the goal. It must be understood, however, that while this is true, a high level of conditioning would serve to contribute even more to your experience. It might also be suggested here that this principle of desire could legitimately be extended to all forms of human movement. It has long been recognized that one rarely, if ever, uses all of one's potential and that sheer willpower can turn failure into success.

To express an idea a dance may be a vigorous, demanding, exciting creation or it may be a lazy, relaxed, or "tired" performance. The diverse nature of the activity suggests that a high level of conditioning is desirable even though it may not be absolutely necessary.

Due to the creative element of dance, there are no predetermined postures, no "best way" to express an idea or thought. Thus, you never really know what movement or body position you might wish to assume. It seems advisable, then, to develop a high degree of strength in all major muscle groups and a wide range of flexibility in major body joints.

Sustained or vigorous dances require a high level of circulo-respiratory endurance. It would be unfortunate to have an idea and the strength and flexibility to express it through movement, only to find that you lack the circulorespiratory endurance necessary to convey the idea through the dance.

The role of relaxation should be viewed as a relative one — relative to the particular movement used for expression. There are times when you will want to express an idea with tense movements, but there will also be times when loose, free, relaxed movements seem most appropriate. Thus, you will want to develop skills of conscious relaxation so that they can be utilized at will.

Golf

Skilled performance in golf demands that the participant swing a long club with enough force to drive the ball two hundred yards and enough accuracy to keep the ball on the fairway. The force factors result from weight transfer and from strength.

This strength should be developed bilaterally, but special attention must be given to the nondominant side. Golf is one of the rare activities that calls upon the right-handed performer to make maximum use of the left side. The nondominant side is likely to be weaker than the dominant and this can subtly introduce error into the swing. The right-handed novice unconsciously compensates for the weakness on the left side by using the strong right side. You may avoid this error by strengthening the muscles in the nondominant hand, wrist, arm, and shoulder.

Rotation of the trunk and spine increases the potential length of the backswing, thereby increasing the force generated in the downswing and ultimately the distance the ball will carry. Thus, the muscles of your trunk must be both strong and flexible. If you are in good physical condition, this should not pose an undue problem, and you should spend your time learning to coordinate the body rotation with the armswing.

Accuracy results from two basic factors: a consistent well-grooved pendulum swing and a firm stable base of support. The former is predominantly skill, while the latter depends upon strong feet and strong muscles in your inner thighs and calves. Most beginners lack the necessary degree of strength in these muscles and would do well to incorporate appropriate exercises into the specific conditioning program. Remember, inadequate strength in the wrist, arm, shoulder, and trunk muscle groups can cause unnecessary learning difficulties.

In golf, flexibility is only a secondary conditioning factor. A certain amount is needed in the shoulder and in the trunk, but most beginners seem to be adequately conditioned in this respect. It is unlikely that you will need to supplement your general conditioning program with exercises for this purpose.

The same generalization applies to circulorespiratory endurance. To be sure, the walk around the course is good for you, but it is not so demanding that you would be fatigued. Perhaps this is true because the golfer is usually able to move at a self-determined pace.

Relaxation is viewed from two different perspectives. First, the golf swing itself should be a smooth, rhythmic, fluid, controlled movement. This can be realized only when you develop a forceful swing without developing unnecessary and undesirable muscular tension. Such tension dissipates energy and force and results in jerky movements. Conscious but controlled relaxation practiced concurrently with recommended movement patterns should help you achieve this desired balance. Second, when played as a recreational activity golf is conducive to relaxation. Perhaps this is true because it is played in an outdoor environment. Take the time to relax and appreciate the natural beauty which is all around you, and in so doing you may find that this is one of the most rewarding facets of the game.

Gymnastic Activities

There are four major events that comprise international gymnastic competition for women: floor exercise, the balance beam, vaulting, and the uneven parallel bars. Such variety suggests that each activity has its own unique characteristics and demands specific physical capacities.

Strength needs will vary somewhat with the event and/or the particular skill being performed. You will need an overall high level of strength in all major muscle groups for successful performance in floor exercise. A high level of leg strength is needed on the balance beam, for the explosive power of a vault as well as for controlled landings from all of the apparatus. Performance on the unevens demands a substantial amount of abdominal, leg, hand, arm, and shoulder girdle strength. Many skills on this piece of equipment place your body in a hanging position so that the weight is borne principally by your hands, arms, and shoulders. When the body is in this posture it is imperative that your pelvis be properly aligned under your shoulders; this kind of alignment demands that you possess considerable abdominal strength. If your abdominals are too weak to hold the correct alignment, the result can be a hollow lower back and a stretched abdominal wall. This potential problem cannot be overemphasized because it is not limited to the unevens. Actually, many body positions assumed by the gymnast encourage this undesirable hollow lower back. Thus, it is preferable to begin strengthening abdominal muscles before participating in gymnastic activities. It is imperative to begin them by the time you begin to participate.

The function of flexibility in free exercise performance cannot be overstated, since this is the quality that lends grace and beauty to the overall movement patterns. Flexibility, especially in the hip joint, also makes a significant contribution to learning skills on the balance beam because smooth, graceful movements are so important here. This capacity is also necessary when learning to vault or perform on the bars. As a gymnastic performer you will always want to emphasize flexibility exercises in your specific conditioning program.

Circulorespiratory endurance is not related to successful apparatus performance in a predominant way and average levels should suffice for the novice. However, it does play a vital role in floor exercise. Here you are called upon to create routines comprised of tumbling and dance skills. If your routine is made up of very vigorous moves you will find that high levels of circulorespiratory endurance enhance your performance.

Again, relaxation is seen to have a tremendously important contribution to make to successful learning of gymnastic activities. As with all skilled athletic performance, there must be a balance between relaxation and tension in the muscle. But there is still another consideration peculiar to this activity—that of safety. Fear and/or inexperience can precipitate tension which can predispose the learner to accidents. From this point of view, the relaxed performer is the safest performer. There will be times when it may be necessary to call upon your conscious relaxation skills to help you acquire the confidence necessary for safe and relaxed participation.

Skating

Ice skating can be a highly rewarding recreational activity. In addition to providing an enjoyable individual experience, it has a lot to offer as a family pastime. Furthermore, it is an activity that has no age barriers since it is as suitable for the elderly as for the very young.

Your first task as a skater will be to learn to balance on the inside and outside edges of the skate blade. Since the blade itself is only one-eighth inch wide, you can imagine how small the edges are. Achievement of balance on this very narrow base is a matter of posture and leg strength. You must have sufficient strength in the antigravity muscles to hold your body erect while the strong muscles of your leg provide a firm, unwavering support.

You may hear people talk about weak ankles and suggest that they are the source of many learning problems. Actually the tendency to turn the ankles in is usually caused by a poorly fitted boot. If your feet are in good general condition and your boot is properly fitted, it should not be necessary to do additional strength exercises.

Flexibility of the hip joint is an important capacity because a wide range of motion at the hip facilitates the deep bending so necessary to a long stroke. You should also exercise to increase your flexibility in the Achilles tendon (the heel cord), because many skating positions will demand that you assume a squat position. You will soon discover that you cannot assume this posture unless there is a considerable amount of elasticity in this tendon.

Both muscular and circulorespiratory endurance contribute to successful learning for the beginning skater. You may find that continually maintaining balance is tiring but this will be overcome as you increase your muscular endurance. Endurance will become increasingly important as your skill increases because you will experience a desire to skate faster and to skate for longer periods of time.

Relaxation is a final factor that you will need to be concerned about, first, because it is so helpful to learning smooth movement patterns, and second, because it is absolutely essential to learning to fall. Sooner or later every skater falls. This need not be a painful or frightening experience if you are able to relax when you begin to lose your balance. If you become tense and "fight" the fall, you are much more likely to be bruised or injured than if you relax and "give" with the fall. Learning to fall ought to be one of your first learning tasks and you will find this is much easier if you have already learned to relax at will.

Skiing

The accomplished skier has developed the ability to maintain a well-balanced body position over a moving base, while shifting body weight to change directions, and overcoming gravitational and frictional forces to stop forward momentum. Such balance feats as these make specific demands with respect to the development of high levels of strength, circulorespiratory endurance, and relaxation.

High levels of strength in the legs, back, and abdominal muscles will facilitate the development of beginning skills as well as continuing improvement. These strengths will contribute to your performance in several significant ways. First, you will more easily assume the natural flexed position so necessary for balance. Second, you will be able to control your skis. Third, you will find it easier to make frequent adjustments to changes in the level of the skiing surface. Fourth, you will be able to execute the desired changes of direction by making weight shifts and body position changes while maintaining a well-balanced alignment. In addition, you will need better-than-average arm and shoulder strength to ride a tow rope and to use poles properly when climbing or moving on the level. It is also significant to note that skiing injuries frequently result when muscles are not sufficiently conditioned to control the body.

In order to assume the forward lean position it will be necessary to stretch the heel cord and the muscles in the back of the leg. Other flexibility needs should be met through your general conditioning program.

Your circulorespiratory endurance must be sufficient to permit you to enjoy several runs without tiring and to help you adjust to any altitude conditions. You may need to supplement your general conditioning program to increase your circulorespiratory endurance.

Relaxation is encouraged for three reasons. First, it facilitates your ability to adapt readily to uneven skiing surfaces and slopes of varying pitch. Second, if you relax you will be more likely to fall without injury when maintaining balance is impossible (see Skating). Third, you will more quickly acquire the feeling of proper body position and movement.

Swimming

The skilled swimmer is one who demonstrates the ability to perform a variety of strokes at varying speeds and over varying distances with the greatest possible efficiency.

The power derived from the combined arm and leg stroke must be sufficient to plane the body at the surface of the water. Only in this position does the swimmer's body offer the least possible resistance to forward motion through the water. You need a relatively high level of arm, shoulder, and leg strength to repeatedly perform a swimming stroke which will provide this essential body position. It seems important to note that due to the multi-muscle involvement, swimming a variety of strokes will be extremely beneficial to your general body conditioning.

You are likely to find that the power generated in the propulsive phase of the flutter kick will be increased if your ankle flexibility is optimal. Greater backward force can be generated when the foot is held in a hyperextended position during the power phase of the kick. Likewise, the foot offers less resistance to forward momentum when held in this streamlined position. Your general conditioning program should meet other flexibility needs for effective swimming.

Some swimming strokes demand a higher level of circulo-respiratory endurance than others. For example, assuming the swimmer's performance is relatively efficient, the elementary backstroke is basically a restful stroke which makes no great demands on the circulorespiratory system. On the other hand, the American crawl stroke is generally considered a more vigorous stroke, particularly when the swimmer is moving at maximal speeds. In addition, the fine regulation and coordination of breathing required for skilled performance of the crawl stroke will be enhanced if you possess a high level of circulorespiratory endurance.

The element of fear sometimes experienced by novice and beginning swimmers may cause undesirable muscle tension which, in turn, causes movements to be restricted. Practicing relaxation techniques should contribute to the beginner's ability to consciously eliminate this type of tension. The feelings of panic experienced by both beginning and skilled swimmers in particular emergency situations may be either the cause or the result of muscle tension that inhibits the functioning of your body. With respect to effective stroking for kicking, relaxation also plays a critical role. Arm muscles should contract when you are stroking and should relax when you are recovering or resting. Likewise, leg muscles should be contracted when you are kicking and relaxed during the resting phase. Glides provide for a period of relatively complete body relaxation. The same is true with floating. In fact, frequently your ability to float is facilitated by muscle relaxation or inhibited by undesirable muscle tension. Your ability to relax certain muscle groups while contracting others should serve to liberate you from some of the unnecessary obstacles which would prevent you from becoming a skilled swimmer.

Tennis

To become a proficient tennis player you must master several strokes as well as demonstrate superior balance, stamina, and agility.

Strength plays a significant role in the development of powerful tennis strokes. A forceful drive or serve requires strong contraction of the arm and shoulder girdle along with strong muscle action in the legs. The strength in the legs also facilitates both the agility and balance so necessary for skilled performance. The tennis player is constantly making quick starts, stops, and changes of direction. A strong wrist, hand, and arm are prerequisites of a firm grip. Since many women seem to lack this strength, you would do well to begin these strengthening exercises early.

Average overall body flexibility ought to be adequate to meet the demands of smooth movement patterns. It will be necessary, however, to be particularly concerned with the range of motion in the wrist. The forehand drive calls for strong wrist flexion, while in the backhand the wrist extends as the racket comes into contact with the ball. This movement requires precise timing and may not be mastered by the beginner, but you will want to be sure that the necessary physical capacity is developed so that it aids rather than hinders your developing skills.

Circulorespiratory endurance must be highly developed if you are to become a successful tennis player. You must possess the endurance needed to continually move rapidly and change positions as you play balls in every part of the court. Without such capacity you may find that you have superior strokes and serving ability but you consistently lose to a less capable player whose circulorespiratory endurance surpasses yours.

Relaxation plays two distinct roles in tennis performance. First, in the position of "readiness" relaxation is emphasized as you stand in an easy but alert position. Second, masterful drives and serves call for a unique balance between relaxation and tension. The arm swing and the grip must be relaxed enough to permit a rhythmic, easy motion; as contact with the ball is made, the grip must tighten slightly and the wrist must be firm.

TEAM SPORTS

Basketball

A skilled basketball player must possess the circulorespiratory endurance to run for extended periods of time, to start, stop, jump, pivot, pass, and shoot repeatedly without tiring to the degree where performance will be hindered.

Your general conditioning program should provide the means for attaining a level of strength in the major body muscles adequate for good basketball play. It should be noted that strong leg muscles will contribute to your ability to attain maximum height when rebounding, shooting, and jumping for tie balls. In addition, leg strength will be a significant factor in your ability to control body momentum and retain your balance when you attempt to stop or change directions suddenly.

Since no unusual flexibility demands are required for skilled performance in basketball, your general conditioning program should provide you with the range of motion needed in the major body joints.

A high level of circulorespiratory endurance is a great asset to the basketball player. The running, dribbling, and jumping movements that are so vital for good basketball play will probably demand additional circulorespiratory conditioning.

As in any activity, the most efficient player is the one who can consciously relax during the incidental and structured rest periods provided in the game. In addition, there are times when relaxation in specific muscle groups will contribute to the execution of a skill. For example, your fingers should relax slightly as you catch a pass or a rebound; your throwing arm should be relatively relaxed as the ball is released on a hook shot, and your arms should be hanging loose and relaxed as you prepare to shoot an underhand free throw.

Field Hockey

The outstanding field hockey player is one who is skilled in stick handling, is agile, quick, and possesses a great deal of stamina.

Good field hockey play will require strong legs and wrists. It is a game which involves considerable running, stopping, starting, and changing directions. Because this is true, leg muscle strength and endurance will either enhance or inhibit your ability to keep up the strenuous pace required. Since several defensive and offensive strokes require using the stick in a manner which eliminates the backswing and/or follow-through, strong wrists are also a primary requirement.

Your general conditioning program should provide most of the range of motion needed to play skilled field hockey. However, you may need to increase your wrist flexibility. In dribbling and passing, and in some tackling techniques, most of the power is generated by a strong wrist snap; hence, increased wrist flexibility may need to be developed.

A hockey field is one hundred yards long and many of the players on the team will be called upon to run at top speed up and down much of that distance. While the players on the forward line are extremely active, perhaps the backing up required of the halfbacks makes these positions the most taxing of all. Since only the umpire may call "time out," and only in case of injury, equipment repair or replacement, or game interference, field hockey demands a high level of circulorespiratory endurance.

Efficiency of performance is a critical factor in field hockey; hence, the reasons for taking advantage of every opportunity to release unnecessary body tension are quite obvious. In addition, there are many occasions when the receiver should "give" with her stick as the ball touches it. Fielding is cited as a primary example, since this "give" is a necessity in order to completely stop the ball and maintain possession of it.

Soccer and Speedball

Since soccer and speedball are similar in many respects, both games will be considered in this discussion. Soccer is a game involving running and kicking while speedball is a running, kicking, and passing game. The field size, number of players, and their respective positions are identical.

In both speedball and soccer considerable leg strength is necessary due to the fact that running, dribbling, trapping, and kicking play a primary role in successful game play. Other strength needs should be provided in your general conditioning program.

Hip and ankle flexibility should be emphasized for successful execution of the kick-up in speedball. Your general conditioning program should be adequate for other range-of-motion needs. However, it should be noted that your ability to rotate your foot inward and outward to kick and dribble will be facilitated if you have good lateral ankle flexibility.

The fact that speedball and soccer are played on a field approximately one hundred by sixty yards gives some indication that a high level of circulorespiratory endurance is a prime prerequisite to skillful performance. The forwards must be able to cover approximately three-fourths of the length of the field maintaining a steady attack on their opponents' goal. The halfbacks receive little or no rest during each eight-minute quarter.

The "give" necessary in catching any ball is also needed to catch the ball in speedball. As in any performance, the ability to relax contributes to the smooth execution of the skills required in the games of speedball and soccer.

Softball

Softball is a highly organized team game with conditioning needs which differ with the position that you play. These variances are great enough to suggest that physical conditioning needs will relate to the position played.

Strength needs relate predominantly to the arms and legs. All players must have a high level of leg strength to provide the explosive power needed for effective base running. Both the infielders and outfielders will benefit from leg strength also, since there are times when good running power makes the difference between catching or stopping a ball as opposed to letting it get by. The catcher experiences a strong demand for leg strength, since she must assume and hold a crouched position as well as be able to move quickly to a standing position. The pitcher also has a need for leg strength, for it adds power to the pitch. Arm and leg strength are prerequisites for throwing with speed and for achieving distance. Since this is required of all team members, it is desirable to develop a high level of arm and leg strength regardless of the position you play. However, if you are an outfielder, you will find it particularly important due to the distance factor.

Flexibility through the hip joint is an asset to the baseman, who must be able to keep one foot on the base and reach in all directions for the ball. Other team members will not need a flexibility level beyond that developed by the general conditioning program.

Circulorespiratory endurance is not a frequent demand in a softball game but do not let this mislead you, because when the need is there, it is an important one. If you are to be capable of running quickly as well as running around all four bases as the opportunity arises, you must possess a high level of circulorespiratory endurance. Since the game itself does little to develop this quality, you will want to add appropriate exercises to your specific conditioning program.

Relaxation again contributes to the smooth, graceful execution of skills and thus has a contribution to make to the total game. You should also note that it functions specifically in catching skills, since you should absorb the impact of the ball by "giving" with it. Softball gloves have been designed to disperse the force and should be used, but they are not sufficient by themselves. You will need to learn a controlled relaxation pattern to prevent an unnecessary and undesirable "jar" when the ball hits the glove. Relaxation is also an important factor when the need arises to slide.

Volleyball

Volleyball can be one of the less active team sports. As such it can be enjoyed by people of all ages who are in good physical condition. Highly competitive volleyball is considerably more vigorous.

The strength demands relate primarily to hand, wrist, and arm muscles, since the play requires either serving, volleying, setting-up, spiking, or blocking. Your general conditioning should provide you with adequate strength levels although some may experience a need to increase hand (finger) strength.

Flexibility can contribute to your volleyball skill in that an ample range of motion will facilitate returning the ball and reaching those "hard to get at" volleys. However, the level of flexibility developed in your general conditioning program should suffice to meet the demands of the game.

Successful team play depends upon each team member playing her own area of the court. Since this area is relatively small, there is no significant need for extremely high levels of circulorespiratory endurance.

Relaxation again has a vital contribution to make to your skill development. Extreme muscular tension will cause early fatigue and can also impair the accuracy of your serves and returns. Therefore, as you assume the "waiting posture" or as you prepare to serve, volley, spike, or block, you will want to strive for balance between muscular contraction and relaxation.

Summary of Basic Concepts

1. Graceful movement is learned, but the learning is based on body condition.
2. Overweight is usually the result of a caloric intake which exceeds the energy expenditure.
3. Physical activity is a vital factor in weight management because it relates directly to energy expenditure.
4. Women who experience a normal menstrual cycle will benefit from mild to vigorous activity.
5. Successful performance in selected sports demands specific conditioning programs which supplement the general conditioning program.

Chapter 4

EXERCISES FOR SPECIFIC NEEDS

An effective exercise program is necessarily individualized. Each person must determine the type and the amount of exercise that will meet her needs and goals. The general conditioning program should include exercises designed to improve circulorespiratory endurance, flexibility, strength, and relaxation.

Begin by selecting exercises that can be performed accurately at your present conditioning level. The number of repetitions of any given exercise is also a personal decision since suggesting a specific number for you could at best be only a guess. For example, to determine a starting number perform (and count) an endurance or strength-developing exercise until you find it a real effort to continue. Perform that number for a week, possibly two weeks. Gradually and progressively increase the number. When an exercise becomes easy, change to another which is more difficult. For example, when you can do twenty knee push-ups easily, change to full push-ups. At this point you will find that you can perform fewer full push-ups. Do as many as you can and gradually you will discover that you increase the number of full push-ups you are able to perform.

When designing your daily conditioning program personal choice may dictate the order but a recommended sequence is endurance, flexibility, strengthening or toning. Some prefer to finish by tapering off with some relaxation exercises. Others might prefer to follow the relaxation with more endurance exercises.

There is no best time of day to exercise but scheduling a given time each day seems to be more conducive to regulating a program. While research seems to indicate that three exercise periods a week are sufficient to build and/or develop an adequate conditioning level, for many people a daily period is necessary to build a lasting habit pattern.

It may be both motivating and regulating to use an exercise chart in order to keep an accurate record of your progress. This is also a means of patterning your program for the most acceptable sequence.

Finally, before designing your program review the recommendations given previously in the conditioning section of the book (pp 3-5).

Warm-Ups and Circulorespiratory Endurance

1. **Running or Jogging**
   Run or jog in your neighborhood or in a park. Measure a 300-yard distance for a goal. Jog and walk it, and keep track of the time you take. Push yourself gradually to reduce your time or to extend the distance of your run.

   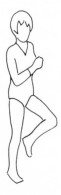

   Figure 3

   When it is not possible to get outside, run in place. Try for the same amount of work (as in the above) by counting your steps or running an equal time. Move lightly on your feet, pushing off with your toes, using your ankles and knees as shock absorbers. For variety lift your knees high and alternate with a high heel kick.

2. **Jumping Jack**
   Jump lightly with a springy push off your toes. Use a vigorous arm swing and stretch your arms high. (See Figure 4.)
   Variation: Use a forward-backward stride jump and change the arm swing position for variety.

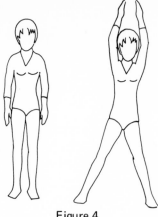

Figure 4

3. **Jumping Rope**

   Jump lightly using the feet, ankles, and knees as shock absorbers. Push yourself, gradually increasing the number of jumps or the length of time you jump.

   Variation: The type of jumping may be changed to provide variety and to increase the difficulty.

4. **Body Swing**

   From a medium squared stance (toes straight ahead, feet 18" apart) swing your arms vigorously up and back as you flex your knees and hips. Gradually increase the amount of flexion and stretch.

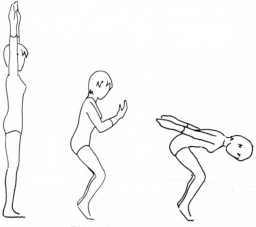

Figure 5

5. **Scissor Jump**

Jump in place, alternate stride forward and back, swinging the arms vigorously in opposition.

<u>Variation</u>: Change the length of the stride, increase the tempo or sink to a shallow knee bend position (no less than 90 degrees) with each jump.

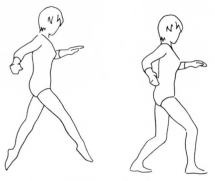

Figure 6

Flexibility (Limbering) Exercises

6. **Legs, Back, Arms**

Stand erect, hips tucked under, abdomen in, and reach to the floor with the hands. Let the weight of the upper trunk help carry you forward and down. Hold the limit of your stretch a few seconds. Shake your legs to loosen them if necessary. Repeat and try to reach further.

7. **Legs, Trunk, Arms**

Assume well-balanced erect standing position. Flex forward from hips, keeping back straight and arms extended in line with trunk. Continue to move slowly as far down as possible, maintaining straight back, arms, and legs. Be sure to keep your head in line with your spine.

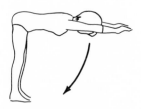

Figure 7

8. **Legs, Trunk, Arms**
   Assume a well-balanced erect standing position. Extend your arms at shoulder level with the palms forward and thumbs up. Maintain straight back, arms, and legs, hold head erect, and move as far forward and down as possible. Hold this stretch position for several seconds.

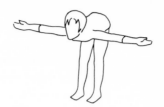

Figure 8

9. **Trunk, Shoulders, Arms**
   Stand erect with one arm straight above head. Reach extended arm over your head, stretching lateral trunk muscles. Make this a pull, not a hip shift. Alternate arms.
   <u>Variation</u>: Add opposite arm pulling across body to increase involvement.

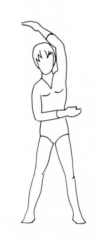

Figure 9

10. **Trunk, Arms, Legs**
    Assume medium stance, arms extended straight above head. Turn upper trunk to side. Reach from hips with back straight, head up. Alternate. As you are able to do this more easily, extend toward the floor. Stretch high when going to opposite side.

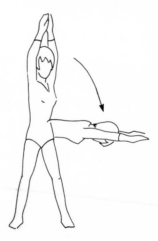

Figure 10

11. **Legs**
    Stand with a long stride, feet pointing ahead, forward leg bent, back leg straight, trunk straight, and arms extended out to side for balance. Press forward over flexed knee as weight is shifted forward. Then flex back knee down as far as possible. Keep heels pressed down to floor. Alternate leg positions and repeat entire sequence.

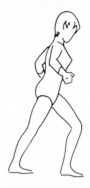

Figure 11

12. **Back, Legs, Arms**
    Sit, legs extended together, back of knees on floor, toes extended, trunk straight, shoulders wide, chin level, arms extended in front of body. Reach forward and grasp the lower leg, holding that position momentarily. Reach farther forward and grasp ankles. Hold. Reach farther forward, hold. Hold body position forward and flex feet. Repeat both positions keeping feet flexed.

13. **Trunk, Legs**
    Assume erect sitting position with arms clasped behind back. Turn upper trunk to leg, stretch forward and down, hold. Stretch straight ahead. Stretch to opposite leg. Repeat all positions reaching forward with the trunk. Hold.

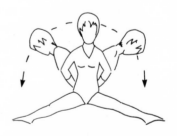

Figure 12

14. Back, Hips

Assume back lying position, maintain a level chin, and pull flexed knee to chest. Alternate legs. Pull both knees to chest. Extend legs and pull alternately and then together.

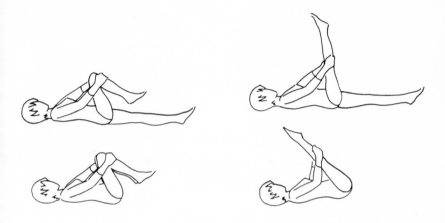

Figure 13

15. Neck

Stand or sit with trunk erect. Rotate head to right and lower chin toward shoulder. Repeat to the left. Return to starting position. Lower ear to right shoulder. Repeat to the left.

16. Shoulder Joints

Take à medium stride, tuck hips under, hold abdomen tight, keep head in good alignment. Circle arms alternately backward. Make movement as big as shoulder joints permit.

17. **Legs**

Take a medium stance. Reach down and as far forward as necessary to touch the floor keeping the legs straight (but be sure knees are not locked). Shift weight gently onto hands and then back on the heels. Rock back and forth.

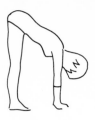

Figure 14

Strength Exercises

Legs: Any of the "warm-up" exercises involving running, jogging, or jumping are good leg strengtheners.

18. **Swing and Hold**

Well-balanced posture, hips tucked under, abdomen tight, head up, arms out at shoulder level for balance. With toes extended, swing leg from the hip as far forward and back as possible with no trunk rotation (at least 10 times to start).

Hold forward for 6 seconds, swing 10, hold back 6 seconds, swing. Alternate legs.

Lift to side 10 times and then hold 6 seconds (no trunk lean). Alternate legs.

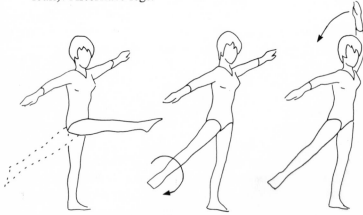

Figure 15

As you lift leg to side, stretch opposite arm over head. Swing leg forward, hold. Slowly bring extended leg around and hold at the back. Return slowly to forward position.

Lift leg to side and circle it from the hip.

When done properly, this exercise works legs and hips actively, tightens buttocks and thighs, uses all trunk muscles, and uses arms and shoulders. Do not touch anything to help maintain your balance; let your muscles do this. If you have hard-to-reach padding on the back of your hips, swing the leg back and hold at an angle that works the area. To increase the work demands on the muscles add some weight for resistance. You can wear a pair of heavy shoes or ski boots for this purpose.

19. **Shallow Knee Bends**
Well-balanced erect pos-ture, square stance, keep heels on floor, do partial bends keeping the knees over the feet. Do not push inward.

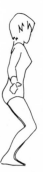

Figure 16

20. **Sitting Slide**
Take a wide stride with toes pointing straight ahead. Keep trunk straight, assume a squat position (not less than 90 degree angle). Shift weight and slide from one side to the other by alternately flexing and extending each leg. Motion should be from side to side, not up and down. Repeat with the toes out at 45 degree angle. (See Figure 17)

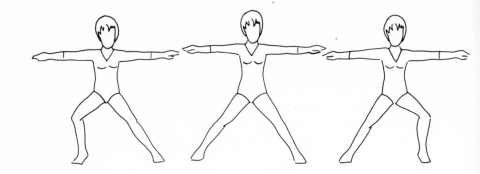

Figure 17

21. **Inner Thighs (Isometric)**
Sit with knees flexed, inner edge of feet together, brace forearm (heel of hand to elbow) between knees. Push knees together as hard as possible. Hold 6 seconds and repeat 5 times.

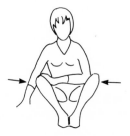

Figure 18

22. **Trunk Lean**
Assume a kneeling position, trunk erect, hands behind lower back. Lean back slowly keeping trunk and head in straight line, return to vertical position. There should be absolutely no arch in the lower back and no sideward bend from the hips.

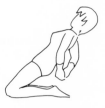

Figure 19

23. Leg Press (Isometric)

Sit facing a partner, legs extended, trunk straight. Place your ankles inside and against those of your partner. (Inside ankles approximately 12" apart). Push out while your partner pushes in for 6 seconds. Place your ankles outside and against those of your partner. Push in while your partner pushes out for 6 seconds. Repeat five times. If you do not have a partner available, use the legs of a stool or chair as a resisting agent.

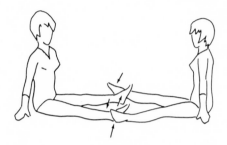

Figure 20

24. Wall Sit

Using the wall as a brace, assume a sitting position and hold for 30 seconds. Increase the length of time you can maintain the position.

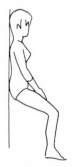

Figure 21

25. Modified Push-Ups

Support the body on the knees (the fleshy part just above the knee, not on kneecap). Place hands wide apart with fingers forward. Keep trunk straight and head up. Lower your body (straight trunk) as far as possible without touching the floor and push up to starting position. Do not lead with the chin or sag in the middle.

26. **Modified Push-Up (Isometric)**

Take the push-up position, shift weight slightly forward moving shoulders ahead of hands, bend elbows slightly, keep trunk straight, hold for 6 seconds. Repeat 5 times.

To increase the difficulty and the work, do the same thing in a full push-up position.

You may also vary this by putting the hands in position with the fingers out, and then with the fingers in. Be sure that the hands are beyond shoulder width so there will be no shortening of chest muscles.

27. **Inverted Push-Up**

Sitting position, legs extended, hands (with fingers forward) behind hips. Lift to a straight trunk position, head in line with trunk. Lower seat to floor. Repeat. This exercise uses the back of the upper arm as well as the trunk and legs. (You will find that this is an area where most women seem to be especially weak.)

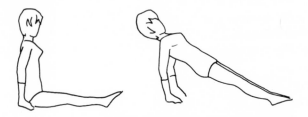

Figure 22

28. **Inverted Push-Up (Isometric)**

Assume the inverted push-up position. Keep the head and trunk in a straight line, bend elbows slightly, and hold for 6 seconds. Repeat 5 times. (When you do this exercise and the regular push-up isometric with the arms slightly bent, you are putting all the work on the muscles. In a straight arm position the body framework does much of the supporting.)

Add difficulty to both push-ups by holding trunk firm and lifting one leg at a time. This taxes all trunk muscles when done properly. (See Figure 23.)

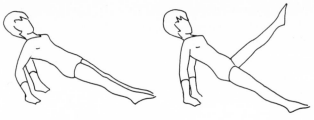

Figure 23

29. Hand and Arm Isometric

Use a soft ball or sponge and squeeze as hard as possible. Feel the tightening through your entire arm and up into the shoulder area. Vary the area tightened by rotating your arm.

30. Arm Rotator

Extend arms at shoulder level, clench fists and rotate arms slowly.

To increase difficulty hold a book and rotate arms slowly.

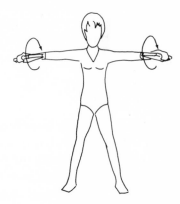

Figure 24

Abdominals

To tighten and firm the abdominal area you must work the diagonal muscles as well as the vertical muscles.

31. Back Flattener

Assume back lying position, knees bent, soles of feet on floor. Tighten abdominals, press lower back to floor, hold 6 seconds and then relax. Repeat at least 5 times.

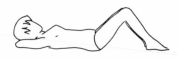

Figure 25

<u>Variation</u>: Hold the lower back flat on the floor by tightening abdominals and slowly push the feet away from the body. When the back starts to arch, pull the feet slowly toward the body. Concentrate on keeping the back flat on the floor during the entire action.

32. **Spine Lift**
    Assume back lying posi-
    tion, knees bent, arms at
    shoulder level with palms
    up. Starting with the tail-
    bone, lift the spine very
    slowly, segment by seg-
    ment. Lift as far as the
    shoulder blades, then
    lower very slowly. Try to
    let down one vertebra at a
    time.

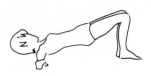

Figure 26

33. **Modified Leg Lowering**
    From a back lying bent knee position, straighten legs extending them toward the ceiling, then lower slowly, stop when the back begins to arch. Bend the knees and circle back to position with legs extended toward ceiling. (If you continue to lower your legs after your back tightens, you are putting considerable strain on the lower back and tilting the pelvis).

    To make the abdominals work harder, hold at a low point for a few seconds but be certain that the lower back does not arch.

    For additional resistance, wear heavy shoes or ski boots.

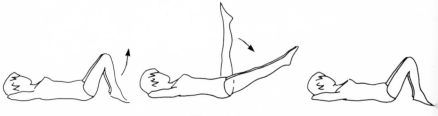

Figure 27

34. Flutter and Cross

Assume back lying position with the arms out at shoulder level. Bend knees and extend legs toward the ceiling. Flutter kick from the hips (18-24 inch span). Lower legs slightly and swing them across each other. Begin with a series of ten flutters and crosses and gradually increase as the muscles permit. Be careful to keep the lower back on the floor.

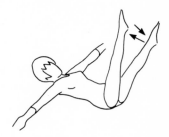

Figure 28

For added resistance wear heavy shoes or ski boots.

35. Trunk Lowering

Assume sitting position with the trunk straight, knees bent, hands behind the lower back, and feet hooked under a heavy object. Keep head and trunk in straight alignment and lower body about 45 degrees, pull slowly back up. Be sure that the back does not arch. Concentrate on doing the work with the abdominal muscles.

Rotate to the right and pull slowly back up. Rotate to the left and pull slowly back up.

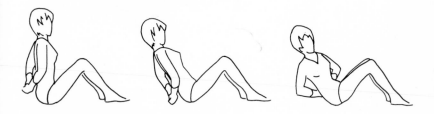

Figure 29

36. **Abdominal Isometric with Partner**
    From a back lying posi-
    tion with legs extended to
    the ceiling, lower the legs
    to a 45 degree angle. Pull
    legs toward the vertical
    against the resistance of
    the partner's hand. Hold
    the angle continuously,
    contracting abdominal
    muscles for 6 seconds.
    Repeat 5 times. Be sure to
    keep back flat against
    floor.

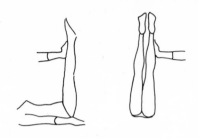

Figure 30

Variation: Back lying position with the legs slightly lowered
to one side. Push to an upright position against the partner's
hand. Hold 6 seconds. Repeat 5 times. Repeat on the other
side.

37. **Leg Press (Isometric)**
    Assume back lying position, legs extended and lowered from
    the vertical, 18-24" apart, ankles together. One partner push
    in and one push out. Hold 6 seconds. Repeat 5 times. Change
    leg positions and repeat. Be sure that the angle of the legs is
    not so great that it puts a strain on your lower back.

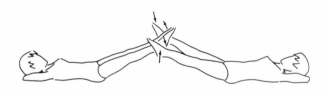

Figure 31

38. Modified Bicycle

Assume back lying position, hips on floor, arms at shoulder level, circle to bring knees back, reach out as far as possible. (The usual bicycling position puts the weight of the body and the force of the action on the neck and shoulders. With the common problem of a forward head, this position is undesirable.)

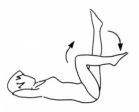

Figure 32

39. "V" Sit

Sit with knees bent, feet flat on floor, palms down on floor behind hips. Keeping trunk in a straight line raise and extend the lower legs to the angle of the thighs and extend the arms at shoulder level. Keep the trunk aligned and try not to rock back.

Variation: Hold the extended position and cross arms and legs back and forth until abdominals are no longer able to hold.

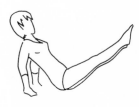

Figure 33

Back

40. Prone Flutter Kick (Lower Back)

Assume prone position, chin resting on hands, lift legs alter-

nately 6 to 8 inches and
hold. Lift both legs and
hold. Flutter kick from the
hips. Keep head down so
the lower back is not ex-
cessively arched. (This exercise also strengthens but-
tock and thigh muscles.)

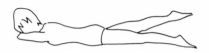

Figure 34

41. **Kneeling Arm Pull (Upper Back)**
Kneel, sit back on heels,
chin down toward knees,
hands on lower back keep-
ing trunk straight. Pull
shoulder blades together.
Do not lift upper trunk.
(When executed properly
this exercise stretches
chest muscles and
strengthens upper back
muscles.)

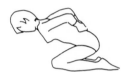

Figure 35

42. **Prone Arm Lift (Upper Back)**
Assume prone position,
arms at shoulder level
with thumbs up and palms
forward. Lift thumbs to-
ward ceiling to pull shoulder blades together. There
will be little movement in
this; the back muscles
should tighten without
pulling anything else out
of line.

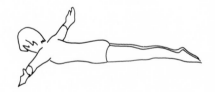

Figure 36

43. Sitting Trunk Straightener

Assume sitting position, knees flexed, soles of feet flat on floor, arms loosely hugging knees. Starting at the hips, slowly straighten the spine until the back is straight. Keep the trunk, shoulders and head in good alignment.

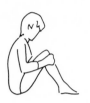 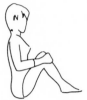

Figure 37

44. Arm Circling

Assume back lying position, knees flexed, soles of feet flat on floor, arms at sides, palms up. Slowly circle arms to position straight above the head by pulling shoulder blades together. Then circle arms back to side.

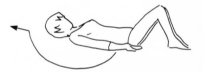

Figure 38

45. Spine Flexor

Sit on a chair. Flex the upper body down as far as possible between legs. Start from the base of the spine, straighten very slowly, and stretch toward the ceiling.

Hips

Many of the exercises listed in other areas are also excellent for strengthening hip muscles. Flutter and Cross, Modified Leg Lowering, Bicycle, Leg Swings, Sitting Slide, Isometric Leg Press are particularly good.

46. Knee Roll

Assume back lying position, knees flexed, soles of feet and lower back flat on floor, arms at shoulder level. Lower the knees to one side, about halfway to the floor. Control the movement by using the hip and abdominal muscles to both lower and lift the knees. Try to keep both hips in contact with the floor. Vary the distance the feet are from the body to determine the position that works the muscles hardest.

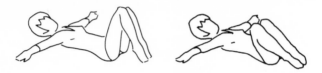

Figure 39

47. Side Lying Leg Lift

Lie on one side with the underneath arm extended to cushion the head and use the top arm to help maintain the side lying position. Lift top leg and hold (use heavy shoe or ski boot for more resistance).

Lift top leg and make small circles from the hip.

Lift top leg against resistance of a partner (resistance must be applied just above knee joint).

Lift both legs, hold, flutter kick

Turn to other side and repeat the sequence.

48. Hip Lowering

Assume inverted push-up position. Lift hips to straight trunk position, rotate hips to right and lower slowly. Return to straight position. Repeat to left.

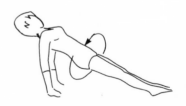

Figure 40

Waistline

Many of the exercises listed for other areas will help to trim the waistline. Any exercise that holds the upper or lower body stationary while the other half rotates against it will help. The knee roll is an excellent waistline exercise.

49. **Windmill**

    Stand with a medium stance, arms extended sideward at shoulder level and legs straight. Rotate upper trunk, keeping arms straight, reach forward and down toward the floor without rotating the hips. Keep the hips stationary and the arms extended and straight. Return to starting position and repeat reaching to other side.

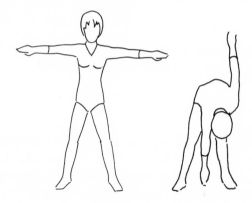

Figure 41

50. **Sitting Windmill**

    Sit with legs extended and apart, trunk straight, arms extended at shoulder level. Rotate arms and trunk as far as possible to right side. Reach forward to the floor. Reach backward to the floor. Move the arms and trunk as one unit.

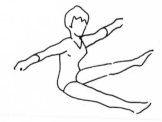

Figure 42

51. Golf Swing
Swinging a golf club properly is a very effective waistline trimmer. It is important to keep the feet stationary throughout.

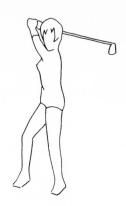

Figure 43

52. Carriage
One of the best waistline trimmers is to stand tall, hold the abdominal muscles tight, and lift the rib cage.

Lateral Trunk

The muscles on the sides of your trunk are used in many of the exercises already suggested and described for strength development. Of particular benefit are the stabilizing effects for the leg swings and particularly the leg swing to the side. Also helpful are any of the push-up or other exercises in which the trunk is held firm and straight.

Bustline

The only exercises that really improve the bustline are those that strengthen the pectoral (chest) muscles without shortening them. The breasts are glandular tissues and are not generally affected by exercise. If there are fat deposits, these may increase or decrease with diet and/or activity. Modified push-ups (both regular and inverted) with the arms wide apart are excellent chest muscle strengtheners. The appearance of the bustline is enhanced by developing strong chest muscles, keeping the head and shoulders back and the rib cage up.

Isometrics

53. Stand erect with hips tucked under arms at shoulder level, elbows bent, hands lightly clasping arms. Tighten muscles and push hands smoothly to elbows (still with light clasp), pull back. Keep head and shoulders back.

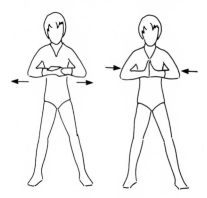

Figure 44

54. Sit in chair, head up, trunk erect, both arms overhead, elbows bent, right elbow in left hand, left elbow in right hand. Pull out, hold for 6 seconds. Repeat 5 times.

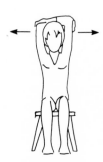

Figure 45

55. Sit in chair, trunk erect, arms overhead, fingers hooked, pull hands apart. Hold 6 seconds. Repeat 5 times.

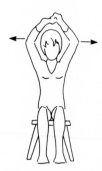

Figure 46

Feet

As with posture, one of the best exercises for feet is continuous correct positioning and usage.

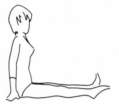

56. In a sitting position, flex and extend your feet.

Figure 47

57. In a sitting position, move your feet in circles from the ankles.

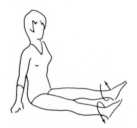

Figure 48

58. In a sitting position "clench" your toes, extend and spread apart as much as possible. Pull toes back as far as possible.

59. In a standing position, put weight on the outside edge of your feet. Curl your toes in and walk. Walk on your heels and then on your toes.

60. Stand with a narrow, square stance. Tighten the buttocks, turn kneecaps out to lift your longitudinal arches. Lift your toes off the floor.

61. Stand on a book, a block of wood, or a step, and curl your toes over the edge. Stretch your toes back.

62. Sit on a chair with your feet on a towel. Pull the towel toward you with the toes and outer border of the foot. Work the length of the towel under your feet.

63. Sit on a chair. Keep your heels on the floor and pick up a marble or other small object with your toes. Lift it to place it on your hand.

64. Sit with your feet resting on the floor. Curl the toes under your feet. Then roll the feet inward so the soles touch each other.

65. Sit in a chair. Roll a bottle or other round object back and forth under your feet.

66. Stand arm's length from the wall with feet in a square stance. Lean to the wall while keeping your heels on the floor.

Relaxation Exercises

67. Start with some overall stretching. Then from a standing position (hips tucked under) swing your arms loosely, one at a time, and let them wrap around your body. Let your head and spine rotate in the direction of each arm swing. Keep the entire action slow. Follow this by swinging both arms in the same manner. Then hang your upper body forward from the hips with your arms dangling. Swing your trunk slowly from side to side and simply let your arms follow your body. Your whole body should feel heavy and loose.

68. This relaxation series involves head and neck action. If this type of neck movement tends to make you dizzy or if you have had a serious neck injury, consult with your physician before doing these exercises. From a standing position (or sitting with legs crossed tailor fashion) with your eyes open, drop your head slowly to your chest and then back as far as possible. Next, move your head from side to side in an ear to shoulder motion. Do not turn or tilt your head but drop it easily from side to side. Again with your eyes open, rotate

your head as far as you can to the right and then to the left. Do this without tilting or tipping the head. Face straight ahead, then turn your head to each side (first right, then left) and drop your chin to your shoulder. Keep the action slow and smooth.

69. From a sitting position with your arms hanging loosely, lift your right shoulder as high as possible and then pull it back and down. Continue to move it in a large circle freely and easily, with the head and arm following along loosely. Make the same movements with your left shoulder and then do it with both shoulders circling simultaneously.

Many relaxation exercises are performed in a supine position. The most advantageous body position is one in which your hips, legs, and feet are slightly higher than your chest. In this position the venous blood flow to your heart is assisted by the force of gravity; hence, your heart rate will decelerate and relaxation will be facilitated.

70. Stretch out on your back with your hips, legs, and feet slightly elevated in a straight plane. At this point you may start with any body area and proceed in any order to do the following: with the arms resting easily at your sides, clench your right fist and feel the tension, the tightness, in the hand, arm, and shoulder. Then relax and let your muscles loosen and spread out. Repeat and concentrate particularly on the loosening phase. Beginning with your palm down, rotate the arm and shoulder until the palm is up. Let the hand slowly flop from palm up to palm down. Follow the same procedure with the other arm and then use both arms together. The amount of time you spend on this will depend on how rapidly you can deliberately relax the area. Do the same thing with your legs; tighten, rotate, and relax. Feel the tension through the relaxation in your foot, leg, and hips. Involve the upper trunk by tightening both arms, hunching (or lifting) your shoulders, and then letting go. Then move to the lower body. Tighten first one leg, then the other, then both legs. Tense the entire body, then relax. Work slowly and deliberately at each step. Concentrate on feeling the extremes of contraction and relaxation.

71. Relax your facial muscles and help to prevent "worry lines" from developing. Starting with the forehead, lift your eyebrows high (your forehead will wrinkle), then relax and feel the forehead smooth out. Squeeze your eyes tightly closed, then quickly release them. Keeping your eyelids closed, move your eyes from side to side, up and down and in large circles. Pucker your lips, grimace, open your mouth wide, wiggle your lower jaw from side to side and down to relax. Tighten all facial muscles as much as possible, then relax.

72. Lie on your back on the floor with arms and legs extended so that your body resembles a large "X." Stretch one arm, hand, and the fingers while keeping the rest of the body as loose as possible. Try to distinguish between feelings of tension in the fingers, hands, and arm and the relaxation in the rest of your body. Then quickly release the stretched arm as you would a stretched rubber band and feel the slackness. Repeat this procedure with the other arm. Then with each leg. Each time feel both the stretch and the release. Finally stretch then relax the entire body.

73. To achieve a generalized feeling of relaxation, lie on your back on the floor, arms comfortable at your sides, legs stretched out with the knees slightly elevated. Breathe easily, inhaling and exhaling slowly. Feel your head as a very heavy attachment to your body. Feel it sinking heavily into the floor. Feel your forehead parting in the middle with each half spreading out toward the side. Breathe easily and feel the jaw loosen and drop as the lips part slightly. Feel the shoulders falling out to the sides, wide and heavy. Feel the hips spreading outward and sinking into the floor. Allow your knees and feet to roll out slightly feeling loose, very loose. As you rest in this position, all body parts should feel loosely connected and heavy, very heavy.

74. Another aid in achieving more complete relaxation may be discovered in the use of mental imagery. It is important to note that while this approach may be soothing and restful for one person, it could be stimulating and exciting to someone else. It is suggested that you try one or more of the following.

Close your eyes and focus on a single, distant object or scene. Think about waves rolling onto a secluded beach at dusk. Picture a beautiful tree standing majestically silent in a large, empty field. Visualize a boat floating lazily on a still mountain lake. See an endless field of ripening grain rippling in a warm summer breeze. Let your gaze rest on a distant peaceful valley bathed in summer sunlight. Try to recall a time when you have been at complete peace with yourself and reconstruct the scene.

Dysmenorrhea

75. **Billig Exercise**
Stand with left side toward wall, feet together and about 18" from wall, legs straight, place left forearm against wall at shoulder height. Place right hand against hollow of right hip, tuck pelvis. Using heel of right hand push hips diagonally forward toward wall. Feel the stretch in the pelvic girdle. Perform exercise three times on each side daily except during menstrual period.

76. **Abdominal Pumping**
Back lying position with knees and hips flexed and feet flat on floor. Push lower back against floor by contracting abdominal muscles. Relax abdominal muscles and arch lower back. Repeat exercise rhythmically fifteen to twenty times.

77. **Golub Exercise**
Stand with a medium stance, arms extended sideward at shoulder level and legs straight. Rotate trunk to left, swing right arm diagonally across your body and touch the left toe. Return to standing position. Rotate trunk to right, swing left arm diagonally across your body and touch the right toe. Return to standing position. Repeat four times, twice daily.

Part II

POSTURE

Chapter 5

INTRODUCTION

Posture as a Personal Characteristic

Have you ever considered the fact that you have only one chance to make a *first* impression? Thereafter, people will see you in light of that first impression. Obviously then, this first image is important. How do you suppose you appear to others? How would you appear on television in an "instant replay"? Have you checked your posture in a three-way mirror recently? Much of the impression created by the "replay" or the reflection in the mirror is a function of your posture.

Posture may be defined as your body carriage; the manner in which you align your body segments when standing, walking, sitting, working, or playing. Whatever your personal manner of carrying your body, you may be sure that it is one of your most conspicuous and personal characteristics. Fortunately, this trait can be aesthetically pleasing; it can suggest vitality, security, assurance, and a positive self-image—an impression all of us would like to convey to others.

The organic or physiological values of well-balanced alignment are not yet clearly understood. In fact, most research indicates that there may not be organic benefits. Nonetheless, this does not negate the obvious contribution to efficient movement and the aesthetic values of well-balanced posture.

Developing Postural Habits

Your posture and appearance reflect the good or bad habits you have been developing for years. When you appraise your posture you may find that your alignment is basically well-balanced. If this is the case, then your primary concern will be with maintaining good alignment with the least amount of energy expenditure. If, on the other hand, your appraisal discloses that your posture leaves much to be desired, you must begin to replace poor (inefficient) habits with correct (efficient) ones. This effort will involve breaking old habits and establishing new ones. Any behavioral change (learning) is contingent upon knowledge, but establishing well-balanced alignment also demands serious, persistent effort and time. It is important that you understand this before you begin to work on postural corrections.

Some of you may discover that you have faulty posture patterns which are not the result of bad habits, but rather were caused by accident, illness, or inherited characteristics. In these cases it is necessary to turn to medical authorities for help. Consult your physician for appropriate exercises and work through him to alleviate the problem. In the meantime you can be aware that proper selection of clothing, style, and color will often serve to minimize the appearance of the deviation.

From childhood through adulthood we are often told to "stand straight," but we are rarely told what the term means. It is difficult to determine just what straight is and how straight feels. It is quite possible to have a good understanding of your postural faults and even know how to correct them but still find that you cannot readily assume and maintain well-balanced alignment. For most people, the missing link, and the most difficult task, seems to be that of *experiencing the feeling* of well-balanced alignment. But you can experience it. And, having done so, you will have gained an efficient, aesthetically pleasing posture that you can henceforth assume at will.

Summary of Basic Concepts

1. Posture, or the alignment of body parts, is a highly individualized characteristic.
2. An individual's posture has a subtle but profound effect upon the impression she creates on others.
3. Positive changes in posture habits demand serious, consistent effort and time.
4. Structural posture deviations are caused by accidents, illness, or inherited characteristics, and their alleviation demands medical assistance and direction.
5. You must work to develop a conscious awareness of the feeling of well-balanced alignment.

Chapter 6

APPRAISAL OF POSTURAL ALIGNMENT

Whether we realize it or not, we are very prone to evaluate some "postures" every day. Likewise, others are very apt to evaluate ours. We do this simply because we tend to observe the people we meet and those with whom we live. These are not likely to be formal appraisals which carefully consider and judge each aspect of alignment. Rather, it is a general impression that we receive or that we give—an impression which subtly suggests that a person is erect or slumped, graceful or clumsy, attractive or sloppy, vibrant or lethargic, confident or insecure. These impressions may or may not accurately reflect the character and temperament of the individual but they are, nonetheless, impressions given. In order to accurately appraise one's posture it is necessary to make a more precise examination of body alignment and carriage than the casual one just described.

You need to observe each of the body segments and note the relationship among these segments. It is most useful to begin an appraisal of body alignment by taking a lateral or side view of one's standing posture. Following this there are other aspects which are best observed from the front or the back. It is the judgments you make about these alignments that form the basis for making further appraisals of your body movements. Because you spend relatively little time in a static (stationary) posture, it is important, indeed necessary, to be further concerned with your dynamic (moving) postures. The real value in appraising your habitual static posture is that it gives an indication of what your dynamic posture will be.

You must have a realistic mental image of your own alignment in order to successfully make posture changes. There are a number of ways to develop this image. In general, the greater the variety of techniques you use, the more realistic your concept of your own posture will be. It may be helpful to have someone evaluate your posture with the aid of a plumb line or another alignment device. But it must be noted that the plumb line is not an absolute measurement; so, it has value only when it is used as a guide or reference point. It is a mistake to use it exclusively as a tool for appraising standing posture. The advantage of the plumb line is that you might get a more objective appraisal but the disadvantage is that you, yourself, have no visual knowledge about the appraisal. For this reason, the posture picture, silhouette, or video tape is widely used. This provides an extended opportunity for you to study and evaluate your alignment. Another advantage of this technique lies in the fact that the picture is very revealing and certainly motivating. There seems to be a tendency toward disbelief of your own postural faults but the picture clearly portrays you as you appear to others. For the picture or silhouette you may be asked to assume what you consider to be your best posture or you may be asked to assume your habitual posture. If the former method is used there is little room for rationalization on your part. By the same token, this may be a stiff, tense, and unnatural posture which does not illustrate your usual carriage. For this reason some teachers will prefer that the picture depict your habitual posture.

Anterior-Posterior Alignment

Anterior-posterior alignment means the alignment of your body as viewed from the side because both the front and back are visible. Your alignment can be checked with a plumb line or with a straight line drawn on a picture. This straight line should run vertically from a point in front of the ankle bone, just back of the knee cap, through the center of the hip, the center of the shoulder, and just in front of the ear. (See Figure 49)

If the overall alignment is relatively straight but slanted diagonally forward or backward you can be reasonably sure that your weight is not evenly distributed over your feet. The line of your silhouette will slant forward if your weight is centered over the balls of your feet (see Figure 50). It will slant backward if your weight is on your heels.

You may find that the line is zigzag instead of straight. This means that one or more of your body segments (usually the head, shoulder, hip, or knee) are out of balance. This zigzag reflects a more

complicated problem than total body slant and will require considerable effort to correct (see Figure 51).

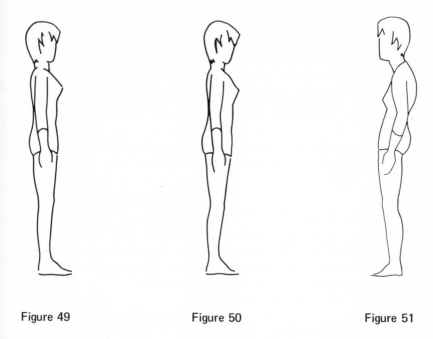

Figure 49   Figure 50   Figure 51

Look first at your head position. The forward head is a most
common fault, yet many people who carry their head in this position
do not realize that they are doing it. The forward head does not
usually show in the fit of clothes or as you view yourself in the
mirror. You may walk with your head down, rest your chin on your
hands to read, sit in a slumped position, or carry things with your
head pulled forward. Many positions and circumstances contribute to
these deviations. Consequently, it is relatively easy to develop a
forward head without realizing it. The results of a forward head will
be more evident in the future than at the present time. As you carry
your head forward you usually exaggerate the spinal curve in your
upper back. The body protects this curve by padding the back of the
neck. The resulting "dowager's hump" is something we all would
choose to avoid. Then too, as the head hangs forward, the chin and
neck tissues are slack, and the sag and wrinkles usually characteristic
of aging will develop prematurely.

The most habitual fault in shoulder alignment is in a forward direction. When the shoulders are forward there is a consequent shortening of chest muscles and stretching of the upper back muscles. Many people are unable to hold their shoulders in correct alignment because of the restriction imposed by shortened chest muscles. This slump does not do much to enhance the bustline. Another disalignment in the shoulder area is a forward slump with an exaggerated rounding of the upper back. Forward shoulders are often observed in conjunction with a forward head and forward tilted pelvis.

Look carefully at your hip position, where it is common to see disalignment. Is there a general slump which accentuates a protruding abdomen accompanied by a hollow or overly arched lower back? Sometimes this is a result of pushing the hips forward (pelvic tilt) or leading with the hips as you walk. However the position of protruding abdomen and buttocks is achieved, the result is aesthetically unlovely and physically undesirable. The flaccid inactive abdominal muscles will pad as excessive fatty tissue is accumulated, and there will be a tendency to continually increase the hard arch in the lower back. And, of course, this position detracts considerably from your appearance in a fitted dress, a leotard, or a bathing suit.

Finally, evaluate your knee position. Another common posture fault results from locking or hyperextending the knees. This action tilts the pelvis forward so that you tend to have a protruding abdomen and an exaggerated curve in the lower back. In addition, a locked knee is highly vulnerable to injury since there is no margin for movement, no room for "give" in the joint. Thus, a sudden pressure on the knee can result in serious and painful injury to the joint.

Lateral Alignment

Your lateral posture is also reflective of your daily habit patterns. By definition, "lateral" means "side," so that lateral posture is evaluated by comparing the right and left sides of the body. This can be done by viewing the total alignment from the front or back. A picture taken from the rear provides opportunity for the most deliberate study (see Figure 52). If you are working alone, you will need to use the front view while facing yourself in a full length mirror.

Start with your head. A sideward tilt of the head could be due to a hearing difficulty or it could be simply a careless habit. If this positioning shows in your check, try to determine the cause and correct it.

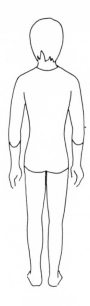

Figure 52

Now look at your shoulders. Is one higher than the other? (See Figure 53.) You may have the habit of carrying books or other loads on only one side of your body. This may result in a low shoulder if you let the weight pull down on your arm. Or it can mean a high shoulder if you tend to hunch against the weight. Try to manage the weight of your loads by using your muscles properly. Check the level of your shoulders in the mirror for practice in the correct feeling. Develop the habit of alternating sides when carrying such items as books, groceries, a suitcase, or a baby (see Figure 54).

Check the hip alignment carefully. Is one hip higher? Or does one hip seem to be more fully padded? You may have a tendency to stand on one foot and shift your weight and/or your pelvis to one side. Or you may push a hip out for use as a shelf to support heavy loads. Check in a mirror. Be aware of the appearance of a difference in hip size. When you continually stand in this position you stretch the muscles on one side. Then any excessive fat padding settles there

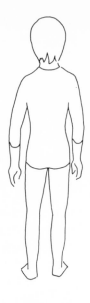

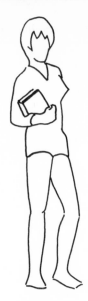

Figure 53   Figure 54

and eventually you develop a noticeable imbalance. The way your skirts fit and hang can be an indication of improper balance. To help prevent or correct this disalignment, tighten your abdominals to keep your pelvis tucked under. Observe your standing position. Stand with one foot forward and shift your weight back and forth rather than from side to side. Holding a standing position is actually more tiring than moving but try to relieve the tension by shifting the weight from the ankles in a way that does not alter good alignment. Also, with one foot ahead of the other, your general appearance is more slim and attractive.

Finally, evaluate your foot position. Ankles which are rolled or turned inward indicate that you are putting your weight on the inside of your feet. This is called eversion. If in addition your toes point out, the condition is called pronation. The weight should be carried toward the outside of the feet and evenly balanced from the heel to the ball of the foot. If you are unable to make this adjustment, it would be wise to consult a medical authority.

Your lateral posture may also be affected by your sitting habits. If you habitually sit on one leg or shift your sitting weight onto one hip you will pull your spine out of line. Because sitting postures have an important and direct bearing on our moving postures, it will be necessary to consider them in greater detail later.

For those who find that their lateral posture is poorly balanced the following additional suggestions should be helpful. Make a habit of using the mirror to be sure your head, shoulders, and hips are level. Then close your eyes and think how the head feels. How do the shoulders feel? How do the hips feel? How does the total alignment feel? Start each morning by making this check on your alignment; then recheck throughout the day at every mirror or reflecting window.

The most important factor in any postural change is the development of a kinesthetic awareness (feeling) for correct alignment. As you begin to make changes and modifications the first efforts will be unnatural, stiff, and strangely exaggerated. As you first try to align the body you may feel "starched." There is no easy or fast way to make lasting corrections; it will take desire, patience, concentration, and continuing practice.

Summary of Basic Concepts

1. Postural appraisal demands a precise examination and evaluation of body alignment.
2. The value of appraising static posture is that it provides an index to dynamic postures.
3. Posture must be evaluated with reference to both anterior-posterior and lateral alignment.
4. The most important factor in any postural change is the development of a kinesthetic awareness, a feeling for correct alignment.

Chapter 7

EXERCISES FOR IMPROVING BODY ALIGNMENT

Now that you have studied your silhouette and identified your alignment problems you can begin to make improvements. Some of the positions and exercises suggested are deliberately exaggerated. This overemphasis should help you to assume and feel the correct position as you practice. For example, the back was not designed to be straight. It has natural curves. But many of you have developed excessive curves which must be decreased. Exaggerating the correction at first by flattening the back should help you to feel and to eventually develop the correct alignment.

Head Alignment

Correcting a forward head will be a challenging task, and will probably require help. What is habitual feels right, while a balanced alignment will at first seem quite peculiar. Your first attempts may be to pull your chin down or to tilt your head up. To assist in correcting the forward head press the neck against the wall and push up with the top of the back of the head. It may help to have someone adjust your head position to be sure that your head is accurately positioned. Close your eyes and think about how the correct position feels.

Shoulder Alignment

When shoulders are carried forward they appear rounded and sometimes slope downward. Too often people with forward shoulders try to improve their alignment by forcing the shoulders way back. This forced position looks as rigid and undesirable as it is. So try instead to experience a feeling of width in the shoulders. Make your shoulders wide and at the same time draw your shoulder blades together. Think, then, how this alignment feels.

Hip Alignment

To help adjust the hip-abdominal area, tuck the hips under as you tighten and pull in and up with the abdominals. This should straighten the tilted pelvis and release the tension on the knees. If you have been a "knee-locker" this change will at first feel as if you have an exaggerated knee bend. With practice the position will become more natural. When you slump in the middle and let your rib cage sag, there is a general thickening in the midriff or waistline. Lift your rib cage and tighten your abdominal muscles. Check your waistline with a tape measure before and after for more conclusive proof. If you cannot achieve the desired effect refer to the exercise section and begin to develop the abdominal strength you need to assume the position.

For an extremely arched lower back, work against the wall by bending the knees and sliding down to a "flat back" position. Slide up and down, maintaining wall contact with the back by concentrating on tight abdominal muscles. You may also use this wall position for work on the upper back by concentrating on pulling the shoulder blades together. Sit down, knees bent, feet flat on the floor, back flat against the wall, arms out at shoulder height, elbows flexed with the forearms against the wall. Hold your arms and the back of your hands as close to the wall as possible, slowly push arms up until they are completely extended, then slowly lower to the original position (see Figure 55).

Knee Alignment

As mentioned earlier, locked knees usually accompany a for-ward-tilted pelvis. The knees should be released from their locked

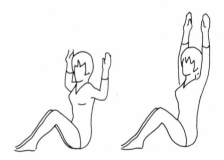

Figure 55

position so that they are held "easy." This does not suggest that the knees bend. Assuming the correct hip-pelvic girdle alignment will be much easier if the knees are easy. By the same token, it is difficult to hyperextend the knees when the hips are in good alignment.

Total Body Alignment

Aligning yourself against the wall is one of the most practical ways of adjusting your posture. Choose an area without obstructions. Stand with your heels three to four inches from the wall. Tuck or roll your hips under and tighten the abdominals to help flatten the lower back. The strengthening of abdominal muscles is particularly essential in maintaining good alignment. There should be only enough room for a flat hand to slip between the lower back and the wall. Hold the hips in this position, draw your shoulder blades together and press back with your head. You are likely to find that at first forcing the shoulders back causes the abdomen to protrude and vice versa but this will become less of a problem as your abdominal strength increases. When you assume and hold this position you will discover that the weight is back toward the heels. Maintaining an erect alignment (feet to head), shift the total body forward from the ankles until you feel your weight equally distributed over the soles of both feet. At first you will probably tend to lead away from the wall with a part of your body (head, hips, etc). Concentrate on feeling the total body alignment, the shift forward from the ankles, and the correct weight distribution. With an increased awareness, practice, and strength development you will be able to control your total alignment.

Another help for practicing total alignment is a "posture stretch" (see Figure 56). Stand in a medium stance with your hands at your sides. As you pull your hands up along your sides, tuck your hips under, pull your abdomen in, and lift the rib cage. Your shoulders should be back and wide, the top of your head stretched up with chin in. Stretch your arms overhead and lace your fingers, pushing palms toward the ceiling. Be sure to hold the tucked position as you stretch. Then bend forward at the hips and hang down. Relax. Repeat. It will take time and practice before you can hold the upright position easily without letting go through the midsection. When it begins to be rather easy, make the trunk adjustments without the arm pull and concentrate on aligning the shoulders and

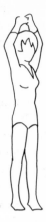

Figure 56

head, or make the stretch upward and then let your arms down gently to your sides.

Walking while balancing a book on the head is sometimes recommended for improving posture. Unfortunately, the ability to balance the book does not guarantee proper alignment. If you use this practice device, be sure that your total body alignment is correct.

Remember that exercises for improving posture will have little influence unless you spend most of your waking day conscious of good alignment. You cannot expect that assuming good alignment for fifteen minutes each day will be sufficient to correct the undesirable habits you have been reinforcing for fifteen years. There are many good exercises that will help you stretch, strengthen, and learn the feeling of position. You will need to strengthen the abdominals, stretch chest muscles, tighten the upper back, and generally strengthen the entire trunk. There is no simple way to permanent correction of poor posture habits. It is a deliberate and painstaking process of unlearning and relearning various positions, feelings, and movements. You will find it extremely helpful to become constantly aware of other people's posture as well as your own. This awareness should serve to trigger continual adjustment and correction on your part. When you observe an extremely good or bad example, let this remind you to correct your own alignment.

Summary of Basic Concepts

1. It may be necessary at first to exaggerate selected body positions in order to "feel" the correction.
2. When correcting alignment for specific body segments, you should concentrate on the feeling of the correction.
3. A desirable total body alignment can be practiced by aligning yourself against the wall or by the "posture stretch."
4. Exercising for postural improvements is not highly beneficial unless you spend most of your waking day in good alignment.

Chapter 8

POSTURES FOR DAILY LIVING

Your living habits demand that you perform countless tasks daily. Within a relatively short span of time you may stand, sit, rise, walk, lift and carry a heavy load of books and set them down. Such tasks are so habituated, so much a part of you, that you may fail to realize that they act upon your body even as you act to perform them. They can have a positive influence and serve to strengthen muscle, increase flexibility, and reinforce endurance, or they can function negatively by placing the body in undesirable positions. When you think of the number of such tasks that you perform daily, it should be evident that it is extremely important to perform these tasks correctly. When this is done they will reinforce your improving posture and help maintain a high level of conditioning.

Sitting Alignment

Incorrect sitting postures can contribute to postural disalignment. A typical "comfortable" sitting pose has the hips forward, back rounded, and head forward. As you recline in this fashion you not only exaggerate the forward head and round upper back, but also put pressure on slack buttocks muscles (see Figure 57). The muscle spread provides opportunity for fat padding and can be a "broaden-

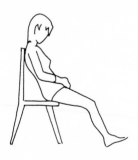

Figure 57

ing" factor. When you depend on muscles rather than using the bony
frame as your sitting base, you may be restricting circulation. Then,
too, as you slide forward in a chair there is very little tone in the
abdominal muscles.

Seating yourself and arising is something you have done hundreds
of times. As students you have spent a significant proportion of your
lifetime sitting. How many of those times have you been concerned
with the way your sitting posture might look to others? How do you
approach the chair? How do you sit in it? If your overall posture
patterns are poor, your sitting habits may range from a carefree flop
and a spread-leg sprawl to a cautious backward reach with your
bottom.

In general, the sitting process should be started from a balanced
position (forward-backward stride) using the strong leg muscles while
maintaining a relatively erect trunk alignment (see Figure 58). If the

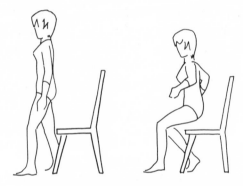

Figure 58

chair is open in front, place the back foot slightly under it with the
back of the leg in contact with the chair. As you sit, flex slightly at
the hips but be sure to keep your trunk straight (from hips to head).
Move well back in the chair so that your bony structure supports you
and takes the force of the body weight (see Figure 59). For a chair
with a closed front, take a balanced stance with your side to the
front edge of the chair. Again, using the strong leg muscles, lower,
slowly turning the hips to sit in the chair. Once seated, keep your
feet flat on the floor if possible. Always reverse the procedure for
rising from the chair. In a deep soft chair, use two moves—come
forward to the edge of the chair and then push up using the leg
muscles to assure a smooth, controlled action.

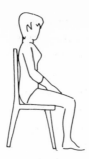

Figure 59

While the preceding general principles apply to all sitting, there is a need to consider some additional guidelines. You must decide what *you* can do attractively. This will be partially determined by your body build, type of clothing, and ability to control your movement. There are some general "watchwords"; knees together, no sharp angles, do not cross legs to bulge muscles, or to restrict the circulation. Remember that the style of dress may restrict you or give you extra freedom. Because someone else looks very attractive in a specific position does not mean that you will.

Because people and chairs come in a variety of shapes and sizes everyone finds it necessary to adjust to some furniture. If the chair is too deep or your legs are short, place a cushion behind your back. In class, use a rectangular briefcase either behind your back or as a footstool.

When sitting to read or write (see Figure 60) follow the same procedure and use your peripheral vision rather than dropping your head over the work and reading or writing "with your nose." Prop your book up or get a book holder rather than bending over a book

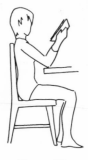

Figure 60

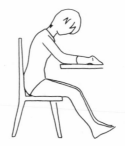

Figure 61

which is lying flat on the desk (see Figure 61). Lean on your arms if you wish, but keep the elbows wide. Do not assume any position that rounds the shoulders, shortens the chest muscles, pulls the head forward, or permits you to sag in the middle. Sitting on a low stool, a floor cushion, or a similar piece of furniture poses more of a problem. Wearing slacks permits considerably more freedom but your movements should be graceful and attractive regardless of your attire. You will need to do some experimenting in front of the mirror. To sit on the floor, move down slowly from a balanced position (see Figure 62). Again, the leg muscles furnish most of the support. Lower the body by placing one hand on the floor at the side of the body. The hand and arm should furnish support on one side as your body approaches the floor. Reverse the procedure to arise, using the hand and arm to assist the legs in pushing the body into an upright position.

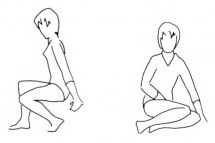

Figure 62

Getting into and out of a car gracefully can pose a problem, especially if the car is small and low (see Figure 63). Get as close to the seat as possible. Keep the trunk erect and lower the body by using your leg muscles. You can do this with either your side or your back to the seat. Move smoothly and avoid leading with your bottom. Getting into the rear seat of a two-door car is a real test. Start with your side close to the car. Facing in the same direction as the car, step in with the nearer foot, bend your knees and slide in, drawing the other foot after you. Weak leg muscles will make this maneuver difficult to accomplish, but it will improve with thought, practice, and increased strength and muscle control.

When getting out of either the front or rear seat of a car you should always lead with the foot nearest the door and reverse the procedure suggested for entering the car.

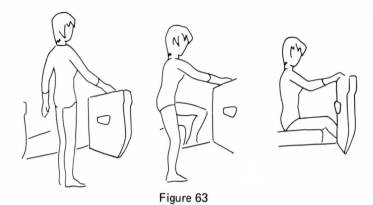

Figure 63

When you drive, take the time to adjust your car seat for height and distance from foot pedals. Use a cushion for your back or to increase your height if this is helpful. Use the seat adjustment to be sure that you are close enough to the accelerator and brake so that your pelvis is not pulled forward on one side, twisting your back. Change the position of the car seat often if you are driving a long distance. This change can be almost as good as a rest.

The way you sit has contributed positively or negatively to your general posture picture, and will continue to do so. People notice the way you sit. Analyze your habits carefully and work diligently to correct those that are undesirable.

Walking Posture

Many times you are recognized from a distance by your walk. Hopefully, it will not be the unattractiveness or oddity of the walk that identifies you. Styles of walking that can be unattractive as well as mechanically inefficient include:

1. A mannish style with forward swinging shoulders and head thrust forward.
2. A waddle walk in which the weight shifts alternately from side to side.
3. A bouncy walk caused by an exaggerated push upward on each step.
4. A toe-out walk with the motion tending to go diagonally forward rather than straight, and with the potential of shifting your weight over the arches rather than the bony framework.

5. A toe-in walk with one or both feet which puts a strain on the knees.
6. An alternate knee-lock walk that gives unnecessary hip action and a jerky bounce.
7. A push-off walk caused by rotating on the ball of the foot. Depending on the direction of the turn you may kick your ankle or splash your legs in wet weather.
8. A disaligned walk with the head forward, the trunk flexed forward from the hips or a hip lead.

It is possible that the styles of walking described may be directly related to foot deformities or abnormalities rather than habit. If there is a question in your mind and you have difficulty correcting your walk consult the proper medical specialist.

To practice correct walking start in the wall position (page 83) with erect alignment. Remember that the total body alignment is vertical so that the weight is distributed over the entire foot. Work on this starting position until you can assume it at will. Now you are ready to meet the challenge of maintaining the alignment while moving.

Since you cannot move gracefully in a completely vertical position, the weight balance must be slightly forward when walking. Again, the adjustment is made at the ankles so that the total body is inclined slightly forward. The mechanically efficient walking motion is a weight shift over the bone structure of the foot. The lead is with the thigh and the weight shift is from the heel along the outer border to the ball of the foot, finally pushing off the great toe. The feet should point straight, or nearly straight, ahead and follow two imaginary parallel lines. The arms will swing easily in opposition to the leg swing. Alignment should be erect and well-balanced. Use your peripheral vision and always keep your head up (chin level).

To increase the speed of walking, lengthen your stride; lean farther forward and push harder against the ground, but keep the movement relaxed, smooth, and controlled. Very consciously maintain your alignment.

When walking upstairs place your entire foot on the tread and, using power furnished by the large muscles of the thigh, push diagonally forward and upward off the ball of the foot. As you step, keep your feet and knees parallel. When descending, the thigh muscles are used in a restraining motion to insure a controlled lowering of the body weight. This strong leg action, with the knees slightly flexed, will give you a smooth, gliding movement as opposed to a bouncy, jerky up-and-down motion (see Figures 64 and 65). When ascending or descending be sure your trunk and head remain in good alignment.

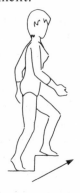

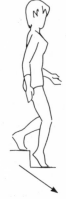

Figure 64   Figure 65

It may be necessary to make some adjustments to varied stair structures or dark and hazardous stairways. If so, remember that the adjustments should be made with the thought of maintaining efficient movement and safe balance.

Standing or walking in high heels requires a deliberate adjustment because heel height tips the weight forward. All too often the unconscious adjustment is a zigzagged one with knees back (locked), abdomen forward, back rounded, and head forward. Make the correct adjustment by maintaining erect alignment and shifting the total body slightly backward from the ankles. When walking, shorten your stride, and it will be easier to maintain the proper adjustment.

In walking uphill, it is necessary to compensate for the incline by shifting the weight forward. The degree of shift will depend upon the slope of the hill. Tilt forward from the ankles rather than bending forward from the waist or hips or leading with the head. Walking downhill necessitates a slight adjustment backward to counteract the angle of the incline. Again, be sure to shift the weight backward from the ankles and maintain an erect alignment.

Always be concerned about efficient daily body mechanics. There may be times when for modeling, photography, TV and/or other interests you will intentionally "strike a pose" or use a special alignment or style of walking. This does not mean that such postures should become habitual and you must learn to resume proper alignment when the "special occasion" is over.

Running

With the emphasis on jogging for conditioning, it is important to review the mechanics of running. All of the action should be forward. There should be no sideward hip swing or leg kick (a typical girl's run). Movement should start at the hip joint with a weight transfer from the heel along the outer edge of the foot, finally pushing off the ball of the foot. As the speed increases there will be more forward lean from the ankles, and only the ball of the foot and the toes contact the ground, or floor. The shock absorbers of the body, the ankles, knees, and arches, should add to the spring and help keep the movement light. The flexed arms should swing easily from the shoulders straight back and forth, in opposition to the foot. To avoid building tension in the arms and shoulders hold the tips of your thumb and ring finger together lightly.

Lifting and Carrying

Your working actions should be graceful, controlled and purposeful, not haphazard and awkward. The ways in which you perform your everyday tasks may serve to reinforce good posture habits and muscle tone or may actually weaken or injure your body and emphasize faulty alignment. Again, it is important to analyze your actions and make definite corrections and adjustments.

It seems advisable to approach any lifting task, light or heavy, by assuming a stooped position. Since most of us tend to be creatures of habit we are most likely to use the approach that becomes a habit with us. Incorrect lifting of heavy weights is responsible for many lower back injuries. If you establish the habit of stooping to lift any object you should lessen the likelihood of sustaining such an injury. The person with a weakened knee joint (or joints) would probably be an exception to this rule. If you have a knee injury obtain medical advice to determine which lifting procedure is best for you.

In any lifting task avoid twisting and turning, since such positions put the back and knees in a vulnerable position for injury. Lifting with straight legs by flexing at the hips puts the strain primarily on the back and is a potentially dangerous action. (See Figure 66.) Properly lifting objects of varying size, shape, and weight involves

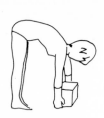 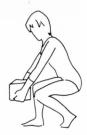

Figure 66   Figure 67

several principles. Get as close to the side of the object as possible.
Assume a forward-backward stride for balance when preparing to
stoop. Lower yourself by bending your knees. Stoop only as far as it
is necessary to grasp the object firmly. Keep the trunk in good
alignment and feel the legs do the lifting as you rise (see Figure 67).
Once you are standing you will need to adjust for the object's weight
by a total body lean in the opposite direction. The slant will
probably be slight, but be sure it is made from the ankle so that erect
total body alignment can be maintained.

If the object has no handle or is heavy, it will need to be carried
in two hands. Hold the stooped position while grasping the object
firmly with both hands. Again, feel the legs do the lifting as you rise.
If you cannot keep your hips under you when lifting a weight, the
load is too heavy; get some help. As you lift or carry the object the
weight of the load must become part of the body as far as balance is
concerned. To carry the object efficiently, hold it as close to your
body as possible.

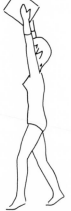 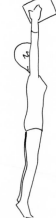

Figure 68   Figure 69

When placing an object on a high shelf use a forward-backward stride and stand near the shelf. Grasp the object firmly and use both hands to lift and place it on the shelf. When reaching for an object from a high shelf, center your weight under the load with a forward-backward stride and keep your knees "easy" but firm (see Figure 68). Assuming a position with the feet together provides an extremely narrow base of support. Hence, in terms of balance, this is a precarious position. (See Figure 69.) When the weight of the load comes onto your hands and arms, be prepared for a controlled "give" so that the leg muscles take the weight. If the object is heavy and your upper arms and shoulder muscles are weak, this may be a difficult, if not dangerous, task, and you should get some assistance.

Pushing and Pulling

There may be times when you cannot get help and an extremely heavy or awkward object can be moved only by pulling (see Figure 70). Keep your body low and use the legs to apply the force in the direction in which you want the object to move. If you can, use a rope to pull the object; the longer the rope, the greater the force you can generate. However, if there is considerable ground or floor resistance to overcome, a shorter rope will be more appropriate.

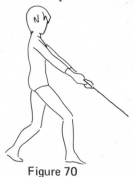

Figure 70

When you have a choice, elect to push rather than to pull or carry. When it is necessary to move a heavy, bulky object such as a chair or davenport, assume a stable crouching position. Keep close to the object and apply your force through the object's weight center. Again use the strong leg muscles to give you power (see Figure 71).

In any endeavor there are very few absolutes, but with reference to lifting and carrying heavy objects there is one. *Never* lift or carry an object which is too heavy for your present strength capacity.

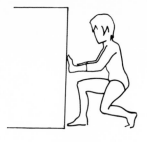

Figure 71

Make it a rule to think before you act. You may well avoid sustaining an injury that could serve as a constant reminder of your carelessness for the rest of your life.

Other Daily Tasks

Besides lifting, carrying, pushing, and pulling there are innumerable daily tasks that are conducive to disalignment. You must be concerned with them because every repetition reinforces unwanted, faulty habits. One such task is hair setting (see Figure 72). Note how the hips and head may push forward, causing a complete disalignment. This is often observable when using a mirror, so check your own habits during this ritual.

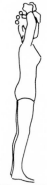

Figure 72

Think about your posture when using a broom, mop, lawn mower, or any other long-handled implement. Avoid the tendency to lean forward rounding the upper back and slumping the shoulders. (See Figure 73.) By maintaining the proper alignment (see Figure 74) you will look and feel better while performing these tasks.

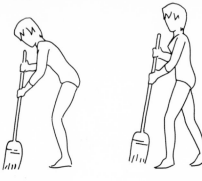

Figure 73   Figure 74

There are some "household hints" that may make your posture efforts easier. Sit to work whenever possible. Try to adjust working surfaces so that you can maintain proper alignment. Be sure that your ironing board is adjustable to your height. A high laundry cart is better than a basket that must be lifted, carried, and lowered. You may not have the opportunity to determine counter and table heights, but you can make height adjustments with chairs and stools. When it is necessary to sit at a table or counter, remember that any trunk adjustment should be made from the hips and not by rounding the back or pulling the head forward.

When you select equipment, do it with the idea of performing your work more efficiently and gracefully. Personalize the "labor-saving" equipment and devices. Be sure that the saving is to your individual benefit.

Summary of Basic Concepts

1. Sitting posture should depend upon the support provided by the muscles, and the bony structure.
2. Your walking posture should be both attractive and mechanically efficient.
3. The ways in which you perform everyday tasks may serve to reinforce good posture habits or may actually emphasize faulty alignment.
4. There are some adjustments that can be made in furniture or household equipment that may make your posture efforts easier.

Chapter 9

WHY THE FEET ARE IMPORTANT

Your feet deserve very careful consideration because they support the standing body, push it off during each moving step, and absorb a myriad of jolts and unbalanced movements. Even in our car-oriented society the average American may walk as much as sixty-five thousand miles during his lifetime. As a student you walk many miles a day (the average housewife walks approximately ten) and give your feet and body innumerable jolts.

The improper usage and care of feet can make your carriage appear clumsy, unattractive. It can also place a tremendous strain on your weight-bearing joints which can lead to unnecessary fatigue and irritation. If your feet hurt or are tired you usually feel "tired all over." Aching and tired feet can reduce your working efficiency and limit your recreational pursuits.

Your foot is composed of many small bones, small muscles, ligaments, and tendons. (One-fourth of all the bones in the body are in the foot.) There are two arches that you need to be concerned with: the longitudinal arch extends from the heel to the toes, and the metatarsal arch comprises the area across the ball of the foot. The arches are "shock absorbers" supported by muscles and ligaments. When the muscles or ligaments are weakened or stretched, the arches can sag. Improper foot usage and/or footwear will do this before you are able to realize it.

The feet take an unbelievable amount of abuse. You may stand and walk with all the weight and force on the arches rather than the bone structure. You may stuff your marvelously adaptable feet into oddly shaped shoes, shoes that offer very little support or the wrong kind of support. The use of ill-fitting shoes may squeeze the toes together with resulting corns, calluses, or bunions. Shoes may not permit your feet to "breathe" because the material of which they are made does not provide for the evaporation of perspiration. Select your footwear carefully. Shop to determine which brand of shoes fit your feet. Determine this by trial, not by observation. Companies manufacture shoes on different lasts or forms. The end product may look the same, but it won't feel the same or fit your foot in the same way. Find a comfortable brand and stay with it. When trying shoes, always walk on a hard nonresilient surface before deciding, because you will not get the proper effect walking on the thick carpeting usually found in stores.

Low-heeled shoes are definitely preferable to high heels. When high heels are worn most of the force of standing and walking is placed on the metatarsal arch with quite painful and sometimes lasting results. Many painful deformities such as bunions, hammer-toes, corns, "pump bumps" on the heel, painful, weak feet, and ingrown toenails can be corrected and reversed with podiatric care by a foot specialist.

In a walking shoe you need more than a thin sole to help absorb some of the force and jar. A thick sole will save wear and tear on the arches. Your selection of hosiery is also significant, because wearing ill-fitting or nonabsorbent hosiery will also contribute to foot difficulties. Specially designed footwear which serves a particular purpose or offers protection is available for most sports. If you expect to spend much time and develop much skill in any given sport, equip yourself properly. Get the advice of experts.

If you have a job that requires spending considerable time standing in one place, be certain you wear shoes that help absorb the force of your weight. Also consider an extra mat or carpet that will provide a resilient surface beneath your feet. Actually, long periods of standing are much more tiring than walking. In walking, the feet are constantly moving, distributing, and changing the pressures, thereby maintaining good blood circulation.

Overweight will tend to produce or contribute to foot fatigue and to possible future trouble because of the increased pressure on the arches. Trouble starts when the weight on the foot is greater than the capacity to bear it. Remember that you have only one pair of feet. It is wise to prevent problems from developing by treating your feet with careful and knowledgeable respect. When a problem develops, consult professional specialists immediately and avoid living with unnecessary discomfort.

Summary of Basic Concepts

1. The feet form the foundation for all standing and most

moving postures and therefore must be firm and strong.

2. The foot is a marvelously adaptable creation, but there are limits to the abuse it can withstand.

3. Selection of proper footwear is an absolute essential of good foot care.

RESOURCE MATERIAL

American Association for Health, Physical Education and Recreation. *Weight Training in Sports and Physical Education.* Washington, D.C.: National Education Association. 1962.

Weight Training in Sports and Physical Education. Washington, D.C.: National Education Association, 1962.

Barney, Vernon S.; Hirst, Cynthia C.; and Jensen, Clayne R. *Conditioning Exercises.* St. Louis: The C. V. Mosby Company. 1965.

Barratt, Marica, *et al. Foundations for Movement.* Dubuque, Iowa: Wm. C. Brown Company Publishers. 1968.

Bowerman, William, and Harris, W. E. *Jogging.* New York: Grosset & Dunlap, Inc. 1967.

Broer, Marion R. *Efficiency of Human Movement.* Philadelphia: W. B. Saunders Company. 1966.

Cooper, Kenneth H. *Aerobics.* New York: Bantam Books Inc. 1968.

Cureton, Thomas K., Jr. *Physical Fitness and Dynamic Health.* New York: The Dial Press, Inc. 1965.

Davis, Elwood C.; Logan, Gene A.; and McKinney, Wayne C. *Biophysical Values of Muscular Activity.* Dubuque, Iowa: Wm. C. Brown Company Publishers. 1965.

deVries, Herbert A. *Physiology of Exercise.* Dubuque, Iowa: Wm. C. Brown Company Publishers. 1966.

Drury, Blanche J. *Posture and Figure Control Through Physical Education.* Palo Alto, California: The National Press. 1961.

Exercise and Fitness. A Collection of Papers Presented at the Colloquium on Exercise and Fitness. Chicago: The Athletic Institute. 1960.

Golding, Lawrence A., and Bos, Ronald R. *Scientific Foundations of Physical Fitness Programs.* Minneapolis, Minnesota: Burgess Publishing Company. 1967.

Howell, Maxwell L., and Morford, W. R. *Fitness Training Methods.* Toronto, Canada: Canadian Association for Health, Physical Education and Recreation Inc.

Hoye, Anna Scott. *Fundamentals of Movement.* Palo Alto, California: The National Press. 1961.

Jacobson, Edmund. *You Must Relax.* New York: McGraw Hill-Book Company. 1962.

Johnson, Warren R., ed. *Science and Medicine of Exercise and Sports.* New York: Harper & Row, Publishers. 1960.

Kiphuth, Robert. *How to Be Fit.* New Haven: Yale University Press. 1956.

Lee, Mabel, and Wagner, Miriam M. *Fundamentals of Body Mechanics and Conditioning.* Philadelphia: W. B. Saunders Company. 1949.

Leighton, Jack R. *Progressive Weight Training.* New York: The Ronald Press Company. 1961.

Lilly, Luella J. *An Overview of Body Mechanics.* Palo Alto, California: Peek Publications. 1967.

Lindsay, Ruth; Jones, Billie J.; and Van Whitey, Ada. *Body Mechanics.* Dubuque, Iowa: Wm. C. Brown Company Publishers. 1968.

Mayer, Jean. *Overweight.* Englewood Cliffs, N. J.: Prentice-Hall Inc. 1968.

_____, and Thomas, Donald W. "Regulation of Food Intake and Obesity." *Science* 156:328-37, April 12, 1967.

Metheny, Eleanor. *Body Dynamics.* New York: McGraw-Hill Book Company. 1952.

Metropolitan Life Insurance Company. *Four Steps to Weight Control.* New York: The Metropolitan Life Insurance Company. 1966.

Morehouse, Laurence E., and Rasch, Philip J. *Sports Medicine for Trainers.* Philadelphia: W. B. Saunders Company. 1963.

Mott, Jane A. *Conditioning and Basic Movement Concepts.* Dubuque, Iowa: Wm. C. Brown Company Publishers. 1968.

Olson, Edward C. *Conditioning.* Columbus, Ohio: Charles E. Merrill Publishing Company. 1968.

Prudden, Bonnie. *Fitness Book.* New York: The Ronald Press Company. 1959.

Prudden, Bonnie. *Teenage Fitness.* New York: Harper and Row, Publishers. 1965.

Rathbone, Josephine L., and Hunt, Valerie V. *Corrective Physical Education.* Philadelphia: W. B. Saunders Company. 1965.

Spackman, Robert R. *Two-Man Isometric Exercise Program for the Whole Body.* Dubuque, Iowa: Wm. C. Brown Company Publishers. 1964.

Steinhaus, Arthur. *How to Keep Fit and Like It.* Chicago: The Dartnell Corporation. 1957.

_____. *Toward an Understanding of Health and Physical Education.* Dubuque: Wm. C. Brown Company Publishers. 1963.

Strauss, Sara. *Here an Inch—There an Inch.* Englewood Cliffs, N. J.: Prentice-Hall Inc. 1964.

The Healthy Life. Special Report by Time-Life Books. New York: Time Inc. 1966.

U. S. Department of Agriculture: "Food and Your Weight," *Home and Garden Bulletin No. 74.* Washington, D. C.: Government Printing Office. 1960.

Wallis, Earl L., and Logan, Gene A. *Figure Improvement and Body Conditioning Through Exercise.* Englewood Cliffs, N. J.: Prentice-Hall Inc. 1964.

Weight Control. A Collection of Papers Presented at the Weight Control Colloquium. Ames, Iowa: The Iowa State College Press. 1955.

Wells, Katherine F. *Posture Exercise Handbook.* New York: The Ronald Press Company. 1963.

Wessel, Janet. *Fitness for the Modern Teenager.* New York: The Ronald Press Company. 1964.

White, Patricia. *Body Contouring, Fitness, and Poise.* Palo Alto, California: Peek Publications. 1966.

INDEX

feet,
    as shock absorbers, 99
    care of, 99-100
    deformities of, 99
    exercises for, 63-64
    overweight and, 100
    selection of footwear, 100
    structure of, 99
    tired and aching, 99
flexibility, 4, 11-13
flexibility exercises, 13, 44-48

Golub exercise, 68

hips, exercises for, 59-60

inherited body type, 3, 12
improving body alignment,
    head, 75, 81
    hip, 76-77, 82
    knee, 82-83
    shoulder, 77, 81
    total body, 83-85
isometric exercise, 8, 9, 50, 51, 53, 56, 63
isotonic exercise, 8

jogging, 42
joint,
    flexibility, 5, 11-13, 15
    structure and function, 11-13

kinesthetic awareness, 79

ligaments, 12
limbering, see flexibility

menstruation, 23-24
mobility, 17
muscle,
    endurance, 4, 7-9, 15